Pathology of Sudden Cardiac Death

An Illustrated Guide

I have chosen to dedicate this book to my wife, Marjorie B. Edwards, and my daughter-in-law, Dr. Terri L. Edwards, for their many encouraging words.

Pathology of Sudden Cardiac Death
An Illustrated Guide

Brooks S. Edwards, MD

Consultant in Cardiovascular Diseases, Mayo Clinic
Professor of Medicine, Mayo Clinic College of Medicine
Rochester, Minnesota

Jesse E. Edwards, MD

Senior Consultant
Jesse E. Edwards Registry of Cardiovascular Diseases
United Hospital
St. Paul, Minnesota; *and*
Emeritus Professor of Pathology
University of Minnesota; *and*
Former Member Section of Anatomic Pathology
Mayo Clinic
Rochester, Minnesota

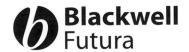

Blackwell Publishing, Inc., 350 Main Street, Malden, Massachusetts 02148-5020, USA
Blackwell Publishing Ltd, 9600 Garsington Road, Oxford OX4 2DQ, UK
Blackwell Science Asia Pty Ltd, 550 Swanston Street, Carlton, Victoria 3053, Australia

First published 2006

ISBN-13: 978-1-4051-2212-2
ISBN-10: 1-4051-2212-9

Library of Congress Cataloging-in-Publication Data

Edwards, Brooks S.
        Pathology of sudden cardiac death : an illustrated guide / Brooks S.
    Edwards, Jesse E. Edwards.
            p. ; cm.
        Includes bibliographical references and index.
        ISBN-13: 978-1-4051-2212-2 (hardcover)
        ISBN-10: 1-4051-2212-9 (hardcover)
        1. Cardiac arrest–Pathophysiology.   I. Edwards, Jesse E.   II. Title.
        [DNLM: 1. Death, Sudden, Cardiac–pathology–Atlases. WG 17 E255p
        2006]
    RC685.C173E35 2006
    616.1′207—dc22

                                                        2005014396

A catalogue record for this title is available from the British Library

Acquisitions: Steve Korn
Development: Fiona Pattison
Set in 9.5/12 Minion and Frutiger by TechBooks
Printed and bound in India by Replika Press PVT Ltd

For further information on Blackwell Publishing, visit our website:
www.blackwellfutura.com

Contents

Preface

What do you do if you are a child of the Depression, have studied and collected almost 30,000 cardiac specimens, and are 94 years old? You write a book to share your experience and knowledge – naturally.

This book is largely the work of my father, Jesse E. Edwards. He defined many of the cardiac conditions that we in clinical cardiology deal with everyday, and in doing so he defined the modern specialty of cardiac pathology. His collection of cardiac specimens has become a worldwide teaching and research tool. Each specimen was carefully dissected, clearly described, photographed, and cataloged. Each specimen held a secret, a lesson for those willing to learn. In discovering the secret of each specimen, physicians and scientists, pathologists, radiologists, cardiologists, and surgeons learned not about the dead but more about the living. In my father's lab, each specimen came alive with the secrets of life and an understanding of disease.

And why does it matter that my father grew up during the Great Depression of the 1920s and '30s? You see, children of the Depression learned not to waste anything – not a piece of string, not a moment of time, and certainly not the lessons for life itself. For each specimen in the collection was the gift of a family that consented to an autopsy with the hope that something could be learned. My father has looked at each specimen as something special; and whether it was collected last month or 60 years ago, there are still more lessons to be learned, secrets to unravel, and a new generation of physicians to educate. For my father, each specimen is in itself a teachable moment.

This project began with the goal of providing a new generation of cardiac specialists with a look at the many processes resulting in sudden cardiac death. Sudden death is now often, although incorrectly, equated with arrhythmic death. As this book illustrates, a host of derangements can result in cardiac death. The focus on pathology provides clinicians the opportunity to see first hand the primary derangements that we often see nowadays only as reflected sound waves, magnetic images, or lumenograms. Sometimes we fail to see anything until a medical examiner's report reminds us of the tenuous nature of life itself. As autopsy rates decline, the opportunity to see first hand and understand disease from the cellular, tissue, or organ perspective becomes a rare opportunity. If a picture is worth a thousand words, this book with its more than 800 illustrations provides the reader with an encyclopedic appreciation for the many faces of cardiac disease and the many causes of sudden death. One cannot help but alter one's clinical practice after seeing the spectrum of pathology resulting in sudden death.

This book in some ways represents the catalog of a collection that will likely never be repeated. While the pathologic processes that we review in this book range from common to unique, the opportunity to see them "in the flesh" is limited.

At 94 years of age most of us are not writing books, but my father is a truly unique individual. His career has spanned the days from before the discovery of antibiotics to the modern-day promise of genomic therapy. He himself has faced many of the challenges of advancing age and benefited from the advances of modern medicine. Through it all, he has maintained a steadfast determination to continue to share his special knowledge and collection so that this precious resource does not go to waste and the sacred promise that somebody will learn from each autopsy is carried forward everyday.

We are delighted to provide this atlas with the expectation that it will provide new insights into the processes of cardiovascular disease, the care of the patient, and the prevention of premature cardiac death.

Brooks S. Edwards, MD
Professor of Medicine (Cardiology)
Mayo Clinic College of Medicine
Rochester, Minnesota
May 2005

Foreword

Sudden death has plagued mankind from time immemorial. One of the earliest descriptions of a sudden death event was reported in Froissart's *Chronicles* in the 14th century, with the first autopsy report of sudden cardiac death ascribed to Leonardo de Vinci in the 15th century. In the 21st century, the Center for Disease Control reported that sudden cardiac death accounted for 63 percent of approximately 730,000 cardiac deaths in calendar year 1999. Sudden death has reached epidemic proportions. During the past few decades the major publications on sudden death have emphasized cardiac risk stratification, electrophysiological mechanisms, and drug- and device-related interventions. Somehow the anatomic and pathologic substrates for sudden death, both cardiac and vascular causes, have been neglected as investigators have focused on disordered electrical function of the heart as the *sine qui non* of this disorder. Fortunately, the link between altered structure and function has been reinvigorated with the publication of Edwards' *Pathology of Sudden Cardiac Death*.

Dr. Jesse Edwards is the pre-eminent cardiovascular pathologist whose contributions span the second half of the 20th century and the beginning of the 21st century. Dr. Edwards is unique in his ability to combine text and detailed photographs of anatomic specimens in case-oriented, clinical-pathological presentations that provide fundamental insight and understanding into the structural and functional alterations of the cardiovascular system involving a spectrum of congenital and acquired cardiac diseases. His first cardiovascular book, *An Atlas of Congenital Anomalies of the Heart* and *Great Vessels*, has remained a classic ever since it was published in 1954. Now, more than 50 years later, Dr. Edwards provides in his latest atlas a compendium of pathologic, physiologic, electrocardiographic, and clinical findings with photographs and text that offer a broad integrated view into the causes of sudden death.

My professional interaction with Dr. Edwards began in 1979 when he, together with Drs. Frank Marcus, Leonard Cobb, and Lewis Kuller, participated as members of the Mortality Committee in our Multicenter Post-infarction Research Study that investigated the factors associated with sudden and non-sudden death during long-term follow-up after survival from acute myocardial infarction. I sat in on several deliberations of this Committee and appreciated Dr. Edwards' ability to integrate clinical data, functional derangements, and autopsy findings, when available, in the identification of the cause of death. The rationale used in the final mortality classification of each patient served the study well. The findings from that study provided the foundation for several landmark drug and device trials investigating therapies to prevent sudden cardiac death.

It has been said that the safe passage into a harbor is marked by sunken ships. Dr. Edwards' *Pathology of Sudden Cardiac Death* is an educational masterpiece directed to pathologists, clinical practitioners, and investigative physicians who are responsible for charting the safe passage of patients through the harbor of life.

Arthur J. Moss, M.D.
Professor of Medicine (Cardiology)
University of Rochester Medical Center
Rochester, New York

Introduction

By far, cardiovascular disease is the leading primary or contributing cause of death in Western society. Cardiovascular death may be sudden and unexpected or may result from known or suspected disease. This book will review and illustrate the multiplicity of mechanisms that can result in cardiovascular collapse and death.

We have chosen to review the topic of cardiac death in the format of an illustrated guide or atlas since we believe the visual picture provides a lasting impression of the fundamental disease states. The cases reviewed in this book span the spectrum from common and ordinary diseases to rare and unusual conditions. By seeing the different states juxtaposed to each other, it is our hope that the reader will appreciate the many conditions that either directly cause sudden cardiac death or provide the substrate for the development of future lethal cardiac conditions.

It is our hope that the reader can quickly assimilate the many different faces of sudden death presented here. As autopsy rates continue to decline, it is our fear that future generations will not have the opportunity to see first hand the fundamental derangements which lead to cardiac disease and mortality. We have attempted to distill many decades of experience into this volume of work in an effort to insure that the experience is passed on to the next generation of scientists and practitioner.

When considering the many causes of cardiovascular death, we will follow an anatomic classification of the primary disorder. The broad categories include the following: coronary artery disease, including atherosclerotic and nonatherosclerotic diseases; myocardial disease; diseases of the conduction system; hypertension; valvular heart disease; metabolic and infiltrative disorders; tumors; disorders of the great vessels, including pulmonary hypertension; pericardial disease; and diseases of multi-organ systems. The illustrative cases in this text come from the autopsies of patients who died in hospital, or from or unexplained death.

Acknowledgments

The photographs in this atlas come predominately from specimens that have been referred from many different pathology laboratories to the Jesse E. Edwards Registry of Cardiovascular Disease at the United Hospital in St. Paul, Minnesota. We wish to thank the families who consented to the postmortem examination for their loved ones in the hope that such an examination could be of service to future generations. We hope this book will be one tangible example of the continuing contributions their loved ones made to the advancement of medicine. The list of physicians who refereed specimens to the Registry is too numerous to mention, but the authors profoundly thank each person who referred material to the Registry.

The authors are grateful to those individuals who processed specimens contributed to the Registry. Among these are Dr. Jack Titus, former director of the Jesse E. Edwards Registry, and Dr. Shannon M. Mackey-Bojack, who is currently leading the efforts of the Registry. Others who contributed significantly to the processing of new specimens include Dr. Karen Kelly, Dr. Susan J. Roe, and Mr. Richard Dykoski.

Mrs. Julie Rooke edited the manuscript to ensure there was a logical order to the many pieces of this project. Her dedication and insightful help were invaluable. Mrs. Jane Jungbauer, former office supervisor of the Registry, participated in the development of the system for specimen and associated material filing and retrieval. Ms. Judith Anderson, current office supervisor, managed the large volume of illustrations and clinical records reviewed for this text. Her knowledge and patience have been deeply appreciated. Ms. Tiffany Dahlberg and Ms. Krista Whitlef also provided outstanding secretarial support for this project.

We wish to acknowledge the support of and encouragement by Mr. Steven Korn of Blackwell Publishing. His enthusiasm for this project allowed it to become a reality. I gratefully acknowledge the expert project management and editorial services provided by Komila Bhat and Fiona Pattison at Blackwell Publishing.

The authors were fortunate for the availability and willingness of Mr. Jack Baldwin to apply his expertise in helping coordinate the development of the manuscript and illustrations, as well as his unfailing good humor, constant support, and guidance. His participation added a pearl to the creation of this manuscript.

I would like to thank Dr. Arthur J. Moss, an admired friend for many years, for providing his thoughtful foreword to the atlas and for his many contributions to the field of cardiology and the prevention of sudden cardiac death.

I wish to acknowledge the specific talents and expertise of Drs. Leonard Schloff, Raymond Gibbons, Allen Brown and Mr. Brad King. Without their help this book would not have been possible. United Hospital Foundation of St. Paul and Mayo Foundation provided the support, environment and necessary infrastructure to allow this project to proceed.

My daughter, Mrs. Ellen Villa, an editor at the *Washington Post*, provided guidance with the development of this manuscript throughout the process.

I wish to thank the following physicians who made suggestions or corrections throughout the compilation of this manuscript. They are Dr. Kenneth Jue, Dr. Milton Hurwitz, Dr. Zev Vlodaver, and Dr. Howard Burchell. Mr. Robert Benassi contributed to this publication by having prepared numerous line drawings that are frequently used in this atlas. He is a valued friend and colleague.

Jesse E. Edwards, MD
St. Paul, Minnesota

CHAPTER 1

Atherosclerotic coronary disease

Atherosclerotic heart disease and its complications continue to be the leading causes of sudden cardiac death in Western society. Cross sections of normal and atherosclerotic coronary arteries are shown in this chapter. The atherosclerotic lesions tend to be eccentric and are made up of accumulations of lipids and fibrous tissue, as well as inflammatory cells. Plaque rupture or localized hemorrhage into the atheroma facing the lumen is the usual precursor to coronary thrombosis. The fibrous tissue separating the site of hemorrhage from the lumen may perforate and lead to thrombosis on the luminal side of the lesion. Once the clot has formed, the thrombus may occlude the lumen of the artery. The thrombus may, with time, undergo organization as it becomes replaced by fibrous tissue and, ultimately, the lumen may become recanalized.

While atherosclerosis is by far the dominant cause of coronary obstruction, there are less common situations that may cause obstruction of the coronary arteries. Such lesions are primarily of the aorta, as, for example, narrowing of a coronary artery and its ostia as it lies adjacent to the beginning of a proximal aortic dissection. Also, in certain cases of trauma to the chest, a resulting laceration may cause obstruction of a coronary artery.

Pathology of coronary atherosclerosis

Cross sections of coronary arteries afflicted with atherosclerosis, two types of lesions are seen: one is purely fibrous, and the other is a pairing of lipid pools and walling fibrous tissue (together these form a "parite") [1]. The combination of collagen and lipid together may be termed *collipid*. In established atherosclerosis, an episodic character to the development of the atheroma is strongly supported. Intimal hemorrhages rarely narrow the lumen but may underlie formation of occlusive thrombi.

Pathologically, calcification in atherosclerosis is a sign of age of the lesion but, by itself, has no direct bearing on the severity of luminal obstruction. The location and shape of the arterial lumen varies in segments with severe atherosclerosis. The lumen may be central or eccentric. In about one quarter of obstructed segments, the lumen appears eccentric and slit-like in prepared histologic sections. Study of distribution of atherosclerotic lesions in all segments of the coronary tree indicates that the segment of the right coronary artery between the marginal vessel and the posterior descending artery is the most commonly involved by atherosclerosis. Second to this site is the proximal half of the left anterior descending coronary artery.

Atherosclerotic aneurysm of coronary arteries

Aneurysm formation affecting the coronary arteries may be caused by coronary atherosclerosis or by an active inflammation of the coronary arteries. The latter subject will be covered in Chapter 2. Aneurysms of coronary arteries secondary to atherosclerosis are characterized by an unusual thickening of the arterial intima of the arteries associated with dilatation of the media. The atherosclerotic aneurysm tends to be isolated and solitary, in contrast to inflammatory causes of aneurysms where there are frequently multiple aneurysms. The external width of the artery is greatly increased in coronary aneurysms, but the lumen is often very narrow. In classical atherosclerosis without aneurysm formation, the effect of the atheromatous deposits causes the lumen to be narrowed; in atherosclerotic aneurysms the lumen is also narrowed but, in contrast, the effect on the media is one of dilatation, and hence formation of the aneurysm.

Sudden death as a first indication of coronary atherosclerosis

Sudden cardiac death may be the first sign of coronary atherosclerosis. While some patients have experienced an emotional or physical traumatic event as a trigger, most cases of sudden death due to coronary artery disease do not have such a clearly inciting antecedent event, and sudden death during sleep is not unusual.

Lecomte and associates [2] reported on the autopsies in cases of sudden death occurring immediately after experiencing emotional stress. Forty-three cases were studied, which included 29 males and 14 females. In 20 cases death occurred during the stressful event; in the other 23 cases, death occurred within two hours of the event. Ninety percent of the patients had no known antecedent clinical history of cardiovascular disease. In spite of this, evidence of previous myocardial infarction was present in 92% of the patients with corresponding coronary atherosclerosis. Cardiomegaly was present in most of the subjects. Acute coronary thrombosis was found in only 8 of 43 cases, suggesting in this series that most of the subjects suffered an arrhythmic death, in the setting of prior silent myocardial infarction.

Myocardial infarction

In patients with coronary atherosclerotic disease, the major clinical risk relates to the development of acute myocardial infarction [3]. There are two frequently used categories of acute myocardial infarction: subendocardial (non-Q wave) infarction and transmural (Q wave) infarction. Subendocardial infarction is frequently associated with coronary atherosclerosis, but usually not acute coronary thrombosis. "Subendocardial" refers to the distribution of the infarction, which tends not to involve the full thickness of the myocardium. While early survival after subendocardial infarction is greater than that observed in transmural infarction, by one year, survival is similar in the two groups. Patients with prior myocardial scarring, transmural or subendocardial, are at risk of ventricular arrhythmias and sudden death. Low ejection fraction (less than 35%) dramatically compounds the risk of sudden death in patients with coronary artery disease.

The second category of acute myocardial infarction is the transmural (Q wave) infarct. The infarction tends to involve almost the full thickness of the involved segments of myocardium. Frequently, preserved myocardium is found near the endocardium of involved segments. Patients with transmural myocardial infarction have a higher risk of developing cardiogenic shock; this may be due to conduction disturbances or valvular malfunction (insufficiency of atrioventricular valves) or simply related to the mass of myocardium lost. In the early stages of acute myocardial infarction, certain pathologic changes may be observed. In early transmural infarction it is common that acute fibrinous pericarditis is seen pathologically as the visceral pericardium becomes inflamed and is covered by a layer of fibrin. Clinically, this pericarditis may present after a silent transmural myocardial infarction and be the only clinical sign of underlying coronary artery disease; the phenomenon is frequently followed by either organization of the fibrin with adhesions or, more commonly, complete healing of the process. Unusually, the fibrin of the associated pericarditis may organize with granulation tissue that may lead to hemorrhagic exudation in the pericardium, a condition that might be confused with rupture of the left ventricle [4]. Rarely the hemorrhagic pericarditis may progress to frank cardiac tamponade.

Histologically, in the early stages of infarction there may be seen the so-called contraction bands, areas of poor staining of the cytoplasm and disorganization. In about 24 hours the site of infarction may be characterized by interstitial leukocytes, namely neutrophils. Associated with the leukocytic infiltration, the infarct has a tendency for early disruption and fragmentation of the myocytes. By the end of the first week the affected myocytes have lost nuclei and are fragmented. The second week is characterized by further fragmentation and disappearance of myocytes. At the end of the first month, the process of postinfarctive removal of infarcted tissue may be nearly completed and scar formation continues.

The gross pictures of acute myocardial infarction reflect the age of the infarct. In the earliest stage there is no recognizable alteration. By one day, the infarcted tissue differs slightly from the normal. During the first week the muscle that is infarcted shows a progressively different quality than the normal areas. At about one week there is a depression between the normal muscle and the adjacent infarct; this depression reflects the early removal of myocardial fibers, leaving only the stroma (capillaries and interstitial tissue). As time goes on, the width of the depression increases and the infarcted muscle yet to be removed is visible as a pale yellow zone. By one month most infarcts will show removal of the infarcted tissue, which will have become replaced by connective tissue. At first the connective tissue is pink and later, as collagen is added, the color becomes gray. At this stage the infarct may be called "healed" by scarring. At the level of the scar the myocardium is thinner than elsewhere.

Nonarrhythmic complications of acute myocardial infarction

Beyond arrhythmic complications, patients with acute myocardial infarction may die from mechanical complications. This subject is well reviewed by Prieto and associates [3]. Large infarctions result in hypotension with both systolic and diastolic dysfunction resulting clinically in an increase in pulmonary capillary wedge pressures. Right ventricular infarction, as well as several forms of rupture of the heart, may lead to lethal nonarrhythmic complications.

Rupture of the heart

Among patients who die from acute myocardial infarction there is a subset of those that develop rupture of the heart [5]. Rupture of the heart is not an unusual finding in medical examiner cases of sudden unexplained cardiac death. There are three anatomical locations for cardiac rupture. The most common type of rupture is that of the free wall, leading to a communication between the left ventricle and the pericardial space. Free wall rupture may be further subdivided according to location: anterior (area of left anterior descending coronary artery), lateral (territory of left circumflex coronary artery), and posterior (territory of right coronary artery or circumflex). The anterolateral region represents the most common location for free wall rupture. In cases of rupture of the free wall, the accumulation of blood in the pericardium occurs rapidly resulting in cardiac tamponade with sudden collapse and death. Early identification of impending rupture may prompt appropriate imaging and potential surgical intervention. Of all the cases

of rupture of the heart, about 85% occur in the free wall. In other cases, rupture of the ventricular septum or left ventricular papillary muscles may occur. Rupture of the ventricular septum has been classified as occurring in either a simple or complex course between the two ventricles [6]. The simple course is characterized by a direct connection between the ventricles. The complex course involves a serpiginous connection between the right and left ventricle, making surgical repair difficult.

In rupture of a papillary muscle, usually multiple heads of a single papillary muscle rupture leading to severe mitral incompetence. Uncommonly, one or only several heads of the papillary muscles are involved in the rupture [7]. In some cases early replacement or repair of the mitral valve may be life saving. In those cases of rupture of the papillary muscle in which a restricted number of heads have been torn, surgical approaches may be delayed [5]. Trauma may cause papillary muscle rupture, as in a case described by Farmery and associates [8]. Additionally, with rupture of a papillary muscle, the laceration of the myocardium may go through the thickness of the left ventricular wall. In such a case [9], rupture of the papillary muscle leads to hemopericardium. Without infarction, blunt trauma such as a deceleration injury from a steering wheel may cause rupture of a left or right ventricular papillary muscle [10,11].

Varying states of healed myocardial infarction

The authors have decided to illustrate several cases of healed myocardial infarction. One group may be subdivided into healed myocardial infarction with either true or false aneurysm. True aneurysm involves an aneurysmal part of the left ventricle with continuity of the myocardium. In a false aneurysm the process is brought about by contained rupture at the site of myocardial infarction [12]. In such cases the site of rupture is devoid of myocardial tissue but instead is made up of scar tissue. The formation of a false aneurysm involves rupture of the left ventricle with retention of some of the hemorrhage by the surrounding pericardium and inflammatory tissue. In the classical case of false aneurysm there is a pocket of blood derived from the left ventricle held in place by the reaction, which may be called the wall of the false aneurysm. In some cases, the wall of the false aneurysm may rupture leading to hemorrhage into the pericardium [13].

Among exceptional cases of false aneurysm is de Boer's report [14], indicating a left ventricular false aneurysm complicating staphylococcal-isolated pericarditis. In a case reported by Lee and Spencer [15] a false aneurysm of the left ventricle was caused by a tumor. And in the case reported by Dubel and associates [16] a huge false aneurysm in the posterior wall of the left ventricle followed resection of a true aneurysm in the same location.

Infarction of the right ventricle

Right ventricular infarction has many ramifications. These depend, to some extent, upon the relative proportion of the right and left ventricles involved in the infarction. In the classical case, right ventricle contraction has been eliminated from contributing to the circulation. The right ventricle then acts in a nonpulsatile conduit between the right atrium and the pulmonary arteries. Generally, patients with right ventricular infarction are older than average and exhibit extensive coronary atherosclerosis [17,18].

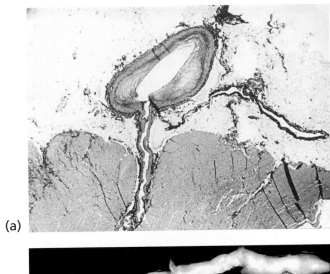

(a)

Figure 1
(a) Epicardial coronary artery supplies subjacent myocardium. An epicardial coronary artery sends a branch, which penetrates the subjacent myocardium. This illustration portrays the source of blood for the myocardium. (b) Endarterectomy of atherosclerotic coronary artery as viewed in gross specimen.

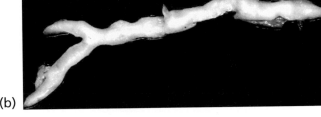

(b)

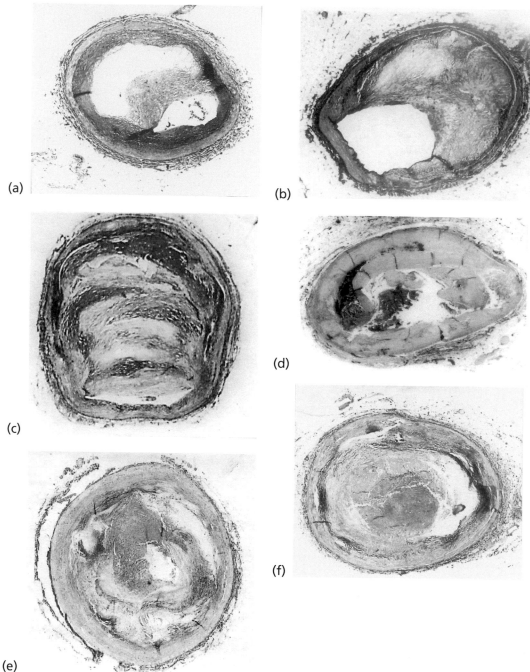

Figure 2 Histology of atherosclerotic coronary arteries.
(a) A classical atherosclerotic lesion. The main substance is lipoid; this is covered by a fibrous cap. The lumen is eccentric and narrow. (b) Atherosclerosis is partly composed of lipoid and partly fibrous tissue. The lumen is narrowed and eccentric. (c) An eccentric atherosclerotic lesion, composed of pairs of fibrous tissue and lipoid. The lumen is markedly narrowed and eccentric. (d) Atherosclerotic lesion with early thrombosis. The fibrous cap over the atheroma has broken. Secondary thrombosis paves the way for ultimate luminal obstruction. (e) Atherosclerotic coronary artery. In the upper half there is a break in the fibrous cap beneath which is thrombus. (f) In the upper zone of the atheroma a break has resulted in a channel containing thrombotic material.

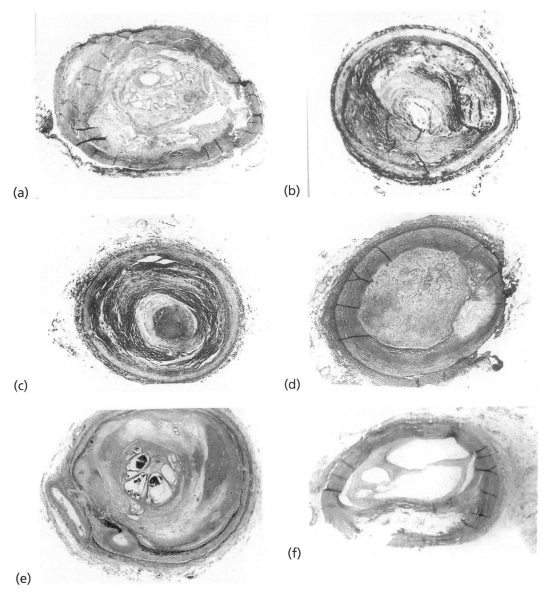

Figure 3 Coronary atherosclerosis, thrombosis, and recanalization.
(a) Atherosclerotic coronary artery. The lumen contains a recent thrombus. (b) In the upper region of the artery an old break is evident. Through this an organized thrombus in the lumen has communicated with the underlying substance of an atheroma. (c) Atherosclerotic coronary artery contains an organized thrombus. The level of this section is above the classical break in the fibrous cap. (d) The lumen contains an organized thrombus. The section of this preparation is away from the site of rupture of the fibrous cap. (e) Organized thrombus showing beginnings of recanalization. (f) Organized thrombus recanalized and represented by multiple channels.

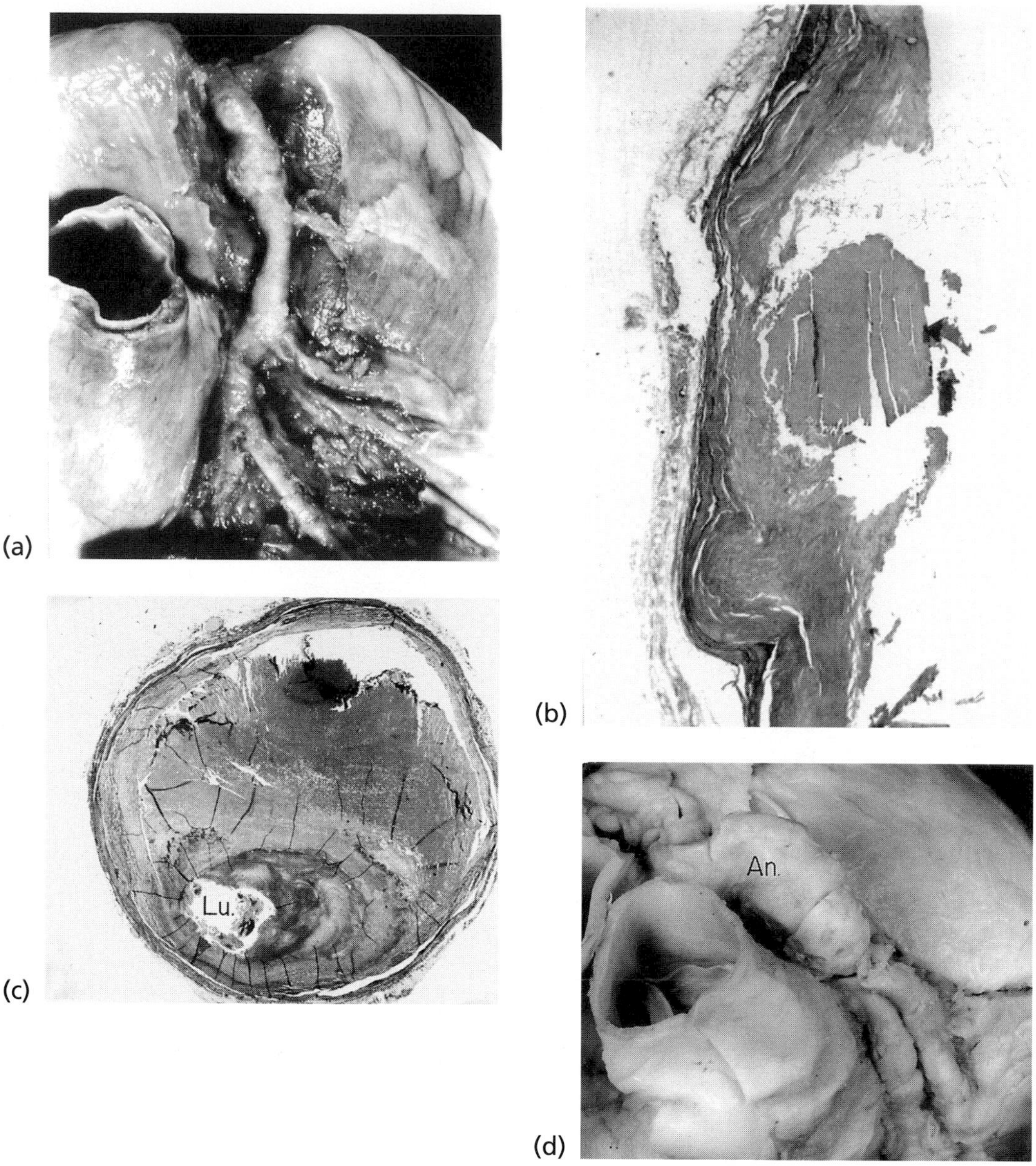

Figure 4 Aneurysm of coronary arteries secondary to atherosclerosis.
Extensive atherosclerosis; the involved coronary artery is widened and associated with deposits of atheromatous material. The lumen of the artery is narrowed. (a) Aneurysmal right coronary artery. (b) Photomicrograph of aneurysmal part of right coronary artery. (c) Cross section of the coronary artery with widening of the wall and deposits of atheromatous material.The lumen (Lu) is marked by Narrowed. (d) Gross view of the involved coronary artery with an Anreurysm (An) involving the proximal portion of the artery. Male, 61 years.
Reprinted with permission from Kalke and Edwards [157].

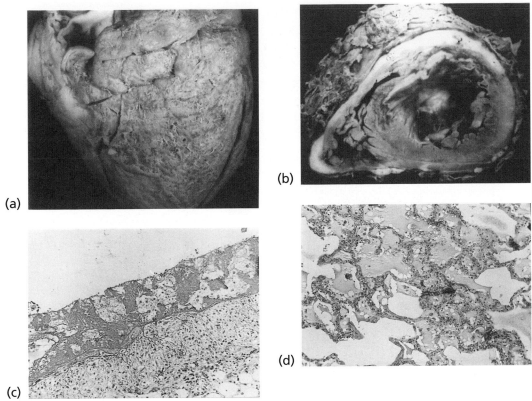

Figure 5 Pericardial exudates and pulmonary edema in acute myocardial infarction.
(a) External view of the epicardium in a case of recent myocardial infarction with sudden death showing fibrinous exudation. Male, 66 years. (b) Cross section of the ventricles revealing a large anterior acute myocardial infarct, surrounded by A which is fibrinous pericardial exudate. (c) Photomicrograph of pericardium in acute fibrinous pericarditis. Male, 66 years. (d) Photomicrograph of lung showing congestion and edema, with fluid in the alveolar spaces.

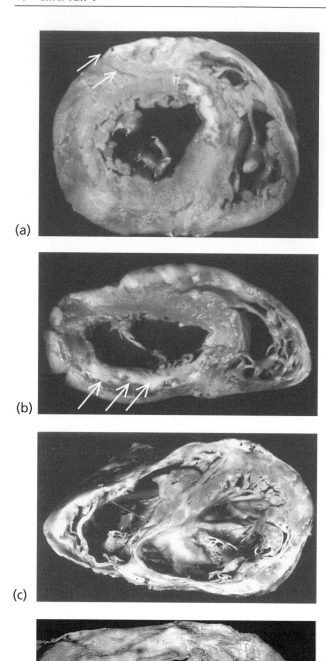

(a)

(b)

(c)

(d)

Figure 6 Examples of acute myocardial infarction.
(a) A large anteroseptal myocardial infarction (arrows). The zone of infarction is localized and may be classified as subendocardial. (b) Cross section of ventricular portion of heart showing discoloration of acute transmural inferior wall myocardial infarction (arrows) leading to sudden death. Female, 48 years. (c) Massive inferior myocardial infarction extending into the right ventricle. Specimen viewed in the following manner: inferior below; anterior above. Male, 54 years. (d) Anterior view of the heart showing extensive acute transmural myocardial infarction. Male, 72 years.

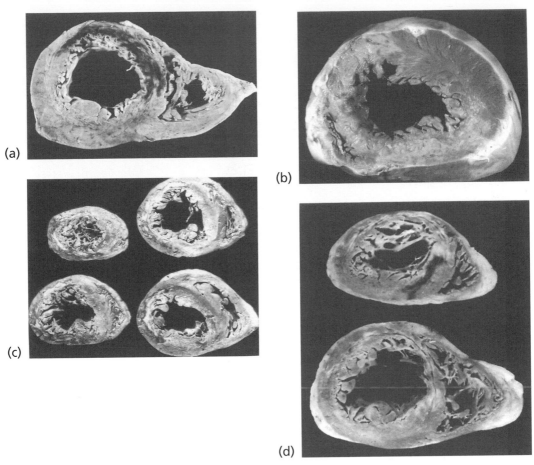

Figure 7 Further examples of acute transmural myocardial infarction.
(a) Broad area involving anterior and septal infarction with intramyocardial hemorrhage; the less distinct discoloration of the inferior wall is evidence of acute inferior infarction. (Viewed from below) Male, 17 years. (b) Acute anteroseptal and lateral myocardial infarction. (Viewed from above) Female, 41 years. (c) Acute transmural myocardial infarction involving almost the entire left ventricle. (d) Acute anterior and posterior myocardial infarction.

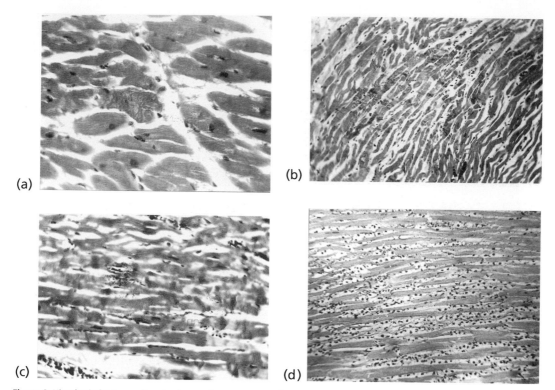

Figure 8 Histologic features of early stages of acute myocardial infarction.
(a) Contraction bands suggesting very early myocardial infarction. Male, 50 years. (b) Contraction bands and thinning of myocardial cells seen in the first hours of myocardial infarction. Male, 78 years. (c) Numerous contraction bands without leukocytic infiltration. Male, 62 years. (d) Leukocytic infiltration in a 2-day-old infarct. Myocardial removal has not begun. Male, 71 years.

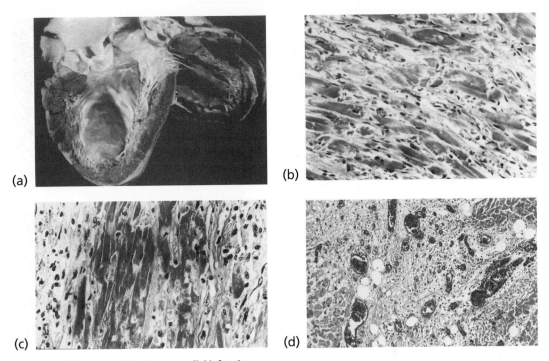

Figure 9 Healing stages of acute myocardial infarction.
(a) Interior of the left ventricle demonstrating myocardial scarring and endocardial thickening in a case of acute myocardial infarction about 2–3 weeks old. (b) Histologic section from a. The section shows a zone of removed myocardium from an infarct that occurred 2–3 weeks earlier sudden death. (c) Histologic appearance of acute myocardial infarction about 9 days old. Some elements of necrotic myocardium are evident; others have been removed. Female, 76 years. (d) Myocardial infarct about 3 months old showing loss of myocardial tissue with remaining vascular stroma.

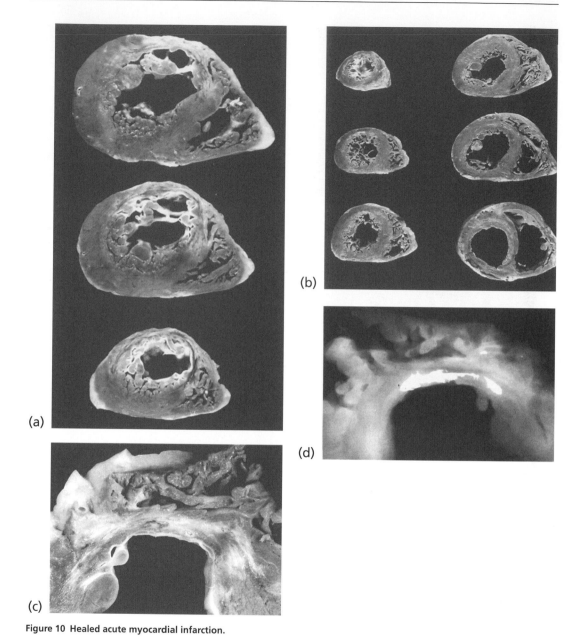

(a)

(b)

(c)

(d)

Figure 10 Healed acute myocardial infarction.
(a) Healed transmural anteroseptal myocardial infarction showing thinning and scarring of the anterior wall. Male,
60 years. (b) Healed subendocardial anterior myocardial infarction. Male, 65 years. (c) Close-up view of healing anterior
transmural myocardial infarction. (d) Close-up view of an old, healed myocardial infarction. The site of infarction is
narrower than in the surrounding myocardium. The infarcted area is partly calcified. Male, 71 years.

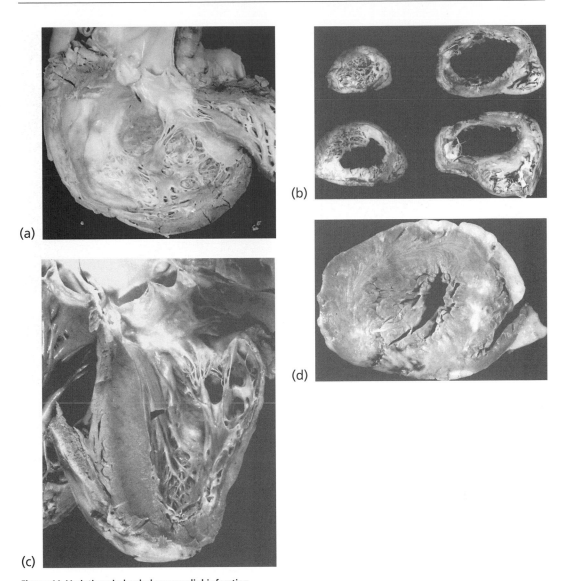

Figure 11 Variations in healed myocardial infarction.
(a) Internal view of the left ventricle. Major ventricular dilatation and thinning of the left ventricular wall due to prior myocardial infarction and subsequent remodeling. (b) Healed circumferential myocardial infarction. There is marked left ventricular dilatation. (c) Healed posterolateral myocardial infarction of left ventricle showing marked thinning of the lateral wall of the left ventricle compared with the ventricular septum. (d) Healed lateral wall and septal infarction and acute inferior wall myocardial infarction with rupture of the left ventricle. Ventricular rupture in a case of previously healed myocardial infarction is unusual. Male, 61 years.

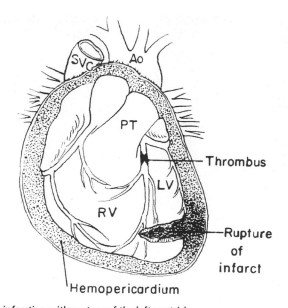

Figure 12 Acute myocardial infarction with rupture of the left ventricle.
The illustration shows hemopericardium resulting from rupture of the ventricular free wall in acute myocardial infarction. This occurs classically from a transmural infarction and, as shown, coronary thrombosis is commonly present.

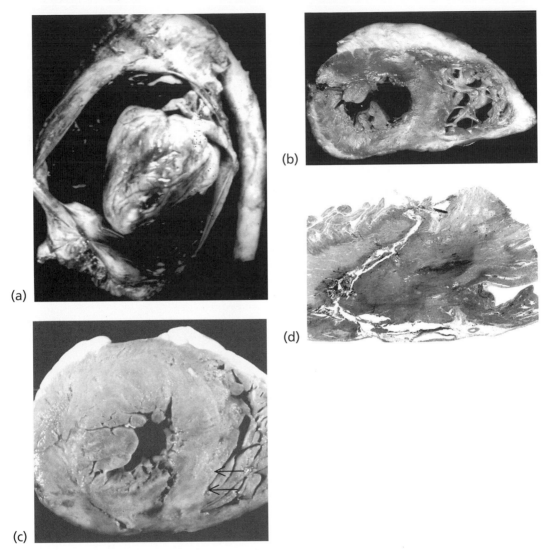

Figure 13 Left ventricular rupture complicating acute myocardial infarction.
(a) Gross specimen of the heart and pericardium. The heart is surrounded by a blood-filled pericardium. Rupture of the free wall of the left ventricle has been followed by gross hemopericardium. (b) Cross section of heart showing acute lateral wall myocardial infarction with rupture of the left ventricle resulting in sudden death. Male, 66 years. (c) Rupture of the inferior wall of the left ventricle arrows complicating acute myocardial infarction. Marked ventricular hypertrophy is present. Male, 72 years. (d) Photomicrograph of specimen seen in c showing the tract of the tear in the wall of the left ventricle. Male, 72 years.

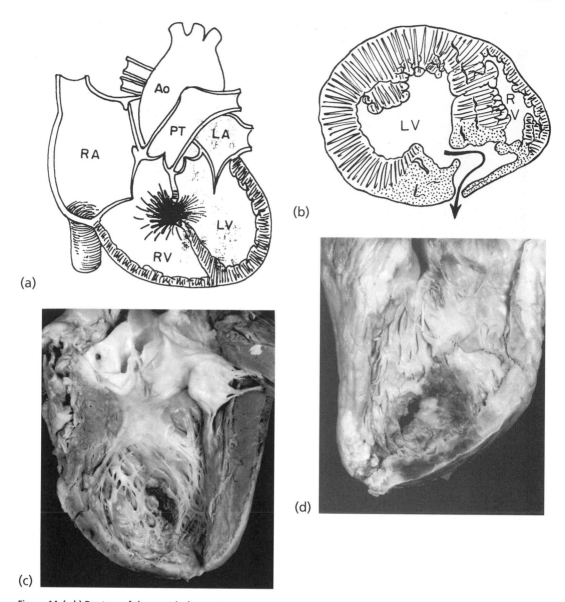

Figure 14 (a,b) Rupture of the ventricular septum.
(a) Illustration demonstrating a simple rupture of ventricular septum with the sudden development of a left to right shunt. (b) Atypical rupture of ventricular septum. The tract of the tear runs from the left ventricle, penetrates the ventricular septum, and enters the pericardium without encountering the right ventricle.
(c,d) Rupture of ventricular septum – simple type.
(c) Interior of left ventricle. A simple tear in the ventricular septum occurring at the apex of the heart is evident. (d) Right side of heart (same case as (c)). Simple ventricular septal rupture following acute inferior wall myocardial infarction.

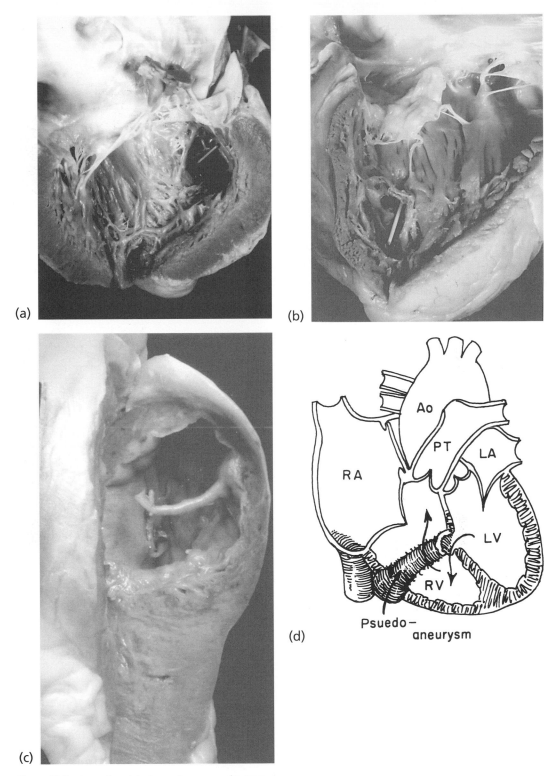

Figure 15 Rupture of ventricular septum – complex type.
(a) Interior left ventricle showing rupture of posterior part of ventricular septum as a complication of acute myocardial infarction. The tract of the rupture follows a serpiginous path. (b) Interior of right ventricle showing the track of the ventricular septal rupture from the left ventricle (probe). (c) Base of right ventricle showing the cavity of a pseudoaneurysm from a contained free wall rupture. (d) Diagrammatic view of complex type of rupture of ventricular septum, including a pseudoaneurysm formed by the tract of rupture.
Reprinted with permission from Edwards et al. [6]

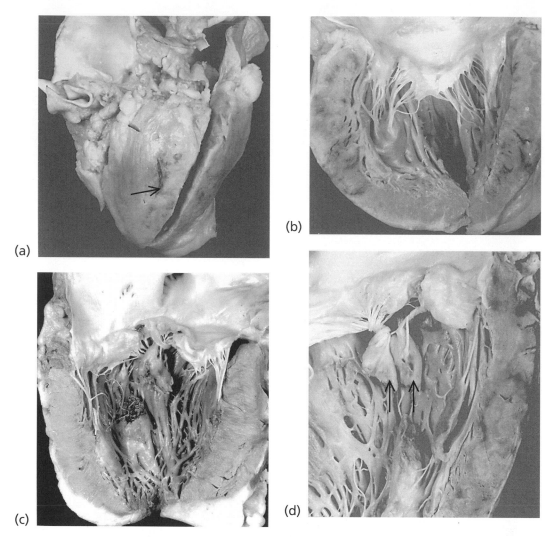

(a)

(b)

(c)

(d)

Figure 16 Acute myocardial infarction with rupture of papillary muscle.
(a) Exterior of left ventricle. Laceration of the anterolateral wall (arrow) showing an exit site from a lateral rupture in acute myocardial infarction. (b) Open left ventricle showing discoloration of upper two thirds of the left ventricle involved with acute myocardial infarction. (c) Total rupture of a papillary muscle due to complication of acute myocardial infarction. There is marked ventricular hypertrophy. Male, 70 years. (d) Total rupture of a papillary muscle (arrow). The unattached portion of the papillary muscle has looped through an intercoiled space. The cut surface of the left ventricle shows evidence of acute infarction. Female, 67 years.

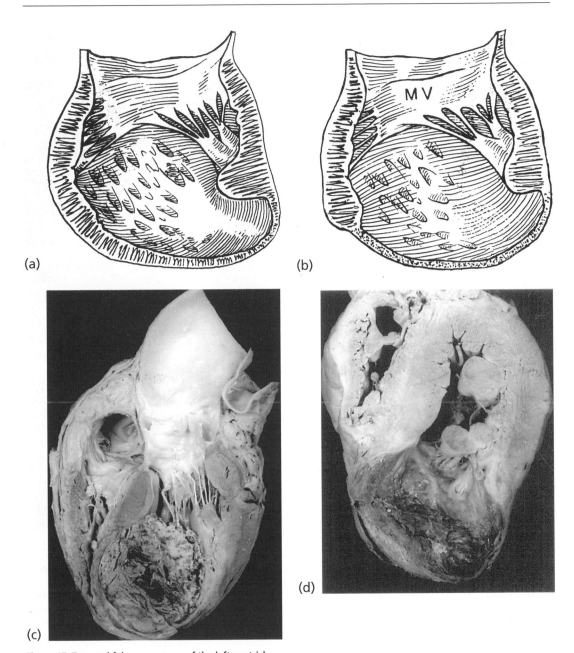

Figure 17 True and false aneurysms of the left ventricle.
(a) Diagrammatic view of true aneurysm of the left ventricle. The configuration is that of a healed myocardial infarction with aneurysm formation. (b) Diagrammatic view of a false aneurysm of the left ventricle. There is loss of continuity of ventricular myocardium resulting in a defect. Beyond the defect, the wall of the cavity is composed of reactive connective tissue but no myocardium. (c) Gross photograph of a true aneurysm of the left ventricle with thrombus in the aneurysm. (d) Gross photograph of a false aneurysm of the left ventricle. Male, 73 years.
Reprinted with permission from Vlodaver et al. [12].

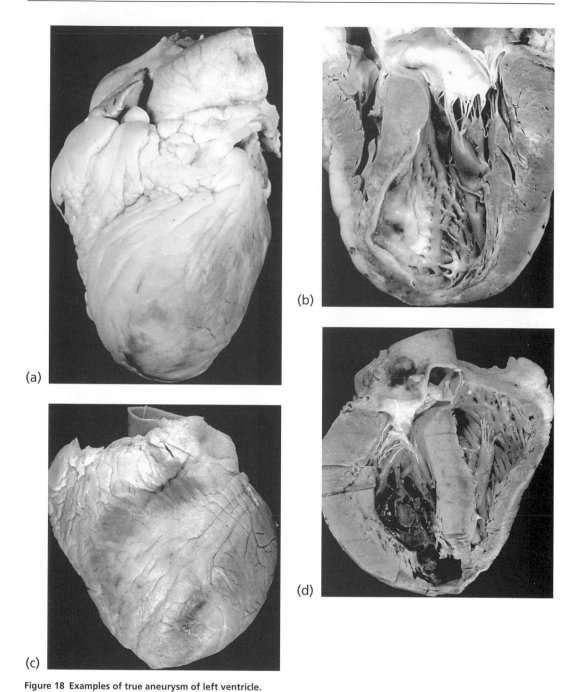

Figure 18 Examples of true aneurysm of left ventricle.
(a) The exterior of the heart shows an apical prominence from a left ventricular aneurysm. (b) Interior of the left ventricle showing healed anterior myocardial infarction with aneurysm formation. (c) Exterior view of the heart showing apical prominence. (d) Ventricles viewed from behind. The early aneurysm of the left ventricle is contributed by partial loss of the myocardium from the left ventricle and ventricular septum.

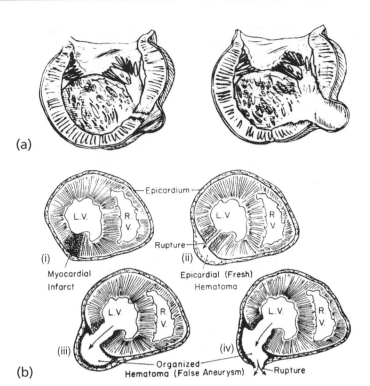

Figure 19 False aneurysm of the left ventricle mechanism.

(a) Diagrammatic representation for the basis of false aneurysm formation. Acute myocardial infarction with rupture (left), and organization of rupture site and associated hematoma (right). These changes lead to an established false aneurysm. Reprinted with permission from Gobel et al. [158]. (b) False aneurysm of the left ventricle. (i) shows the primary rupture site of the left ventricle. (ii) and (iii) show rupture of the left ventricle with restricted hematoma. (iv) shows that the hematoma or false aneurysm shown in (iii) has ruptured, leading to sudden death.

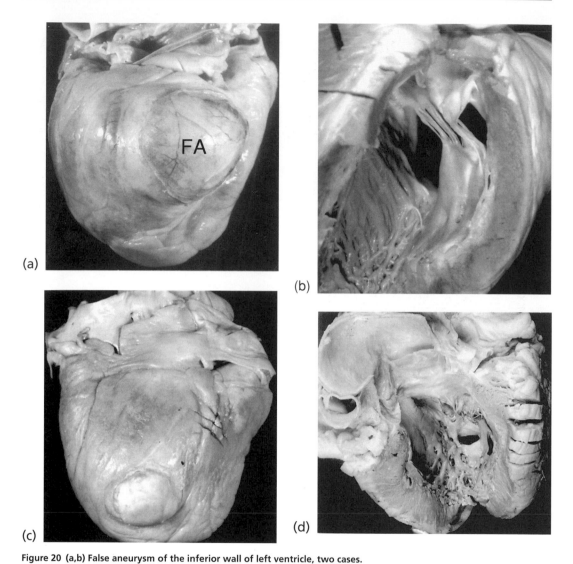

(a)

(b)

(c)

(d)

Figure 20 (a,b) False aneurysm of the inferior wall of left ventricle, two cases.
(a) Exterior of heart showing a deformity at the posterior wall of the left ventricle due to a False Aneurysm (FA).
(b) Interior of left ventricle showing the mouth of the aneurysm beyond a papillary muscle. Male, 69 years.
(c,d) Infected aneurysm of left ventricle.
(c) Heart viewed from behind. Exterior of heart showing deformity of the posterior wall of the left ventricle. (d) Interior of left ventricle showing narrow mouth of the related false aneurysm. Male, 84 years.

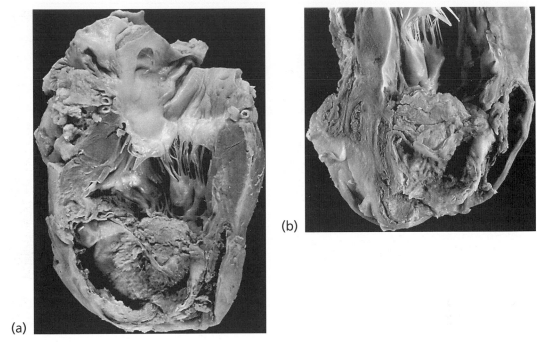

(b)

(a)

Figure 21 Infected true aneurysm of left ventricle.
(a) View of the left ventricle showing an aneurysm at the apical half. The aneurysm is lined by a fibrinopurulent exudate.
(b) Sagittal section of the ventricles showing the infected aneurysm with major cavitation of the ventricular septum and of the lateral wall of the left ventricle. Male, 72 years.

CHAPTER 2

Nonatherosclerotic coronary disease

Anomalies of the coronary arteries

Coronary circulation supplied in part from pulmonary artery

The major anatomic disorder in this category is origin of the left coronary artery from the pulmonary trunk [19]. This condition may result in major complications including myocardial ischemia, myocardial infarction, and secondary mitral regurgitation. A rare example of this anomaly is illustrated in the case of a patient having the left anterior descending coronary artery arising from the pulmonary trunk while the left circumflex coronary artery arises from the right coronary artery, the latter arising from the aorta. This entity may present with an episode of sudden death.

Shunt from aorta to a right-sided chamber

Certain anomalies of the coronary arteries relate to congenital shunts beginning at the aorta and ending in a right sided chamber or vessel [20]. These disorders include rupture of a sinus of Valsalva (aortic sinus) aneurysm into the right ventricle or right atrium.

Coronary artery arising from the "wrong" aortic sinus

A relatively common and potentially important anomaly of the coronary system is that in which a coronary artery arises from the "wrong" aortic sinus [21]; for example, the left coronary artery arising from the right aortic sinus. Some of these patients manifest exertional angina. In cases of this type, sudden death has occurred during or shortly following vigorous exercise [22]. Several cases

surgical intervention has resulted in a favorable outcome.

High origin of a coronary artery

In addition to the origin of a coronary artery arising from the "wrong" sinus there are cases of sudden death in patients with high origin of a coronary artery from the "correct" sinus. Abnormally high origin or acute angular origin of a coronary artery may be associated with sudden death [23].

Aortic dissection causing coronary artery obstruction

Coronary obstruction may occur in the early stage of proximal aortic dissection. This may result when the initial tear of the aorta corresponds to the site of origin of a coronary artery. When aortic dissection compromises a coronary artery, it preferentially affects the right coronary artery.

Injuries to coronary arteries

During cardiac catheterization, the advancing edge of the catheter may penetrate the intima and develop a dissection tract into the media; this results in compromise of the lumen, setting the stage for infarction and, potentially, sudden death. While the literature is replete with accounts of coronary artery dissection or perforations of the coronary arteries during percutaneous intervention, the overall incidence of such occurrences causing major clinical consequences is rare [24].

An often unappreciated complication from cardiac catheterization that may be lethal occurs if the surface of the operator's glove is contaminated with talcum powder. This may lead to delivery of particles of talc into the coronary artery and myocardium.

Emboli to coronary arteries

There are surprisingly many conditions favoring emboli into the coronary arteries. Among these are calcific emboli from calcification of the mitral ring seen especially following surgical replacement of the mitral valve, or calcific particles from calcific aortic stenosis (with or without surgical intervention). In addition, bacterial endocarditis as well as nonbacterial endocarditis may produce emboli from vegetations that develop on valve surfaces. Cholesterol crystals, seen in cases of cholesterol embolism, may affect the coronary circulation. Old venous coronary artery bypass grafts may develop atherosclerosis and lead to distal coronary emboli.

It is not uncommon to find thrombotic emboli to systemic arteries in patients with mitral stenosis. The emboli vary in age from recent to old and well organized [25].

Drugs affecting coronary arteries

Cocaine and other vasoconstrictors may be associated with prominent infiltration of the media and intima by inflammatory cells, resulting in major narrowing of the coronary arterial lumen. This, along with associated coronary vasospasm, may result in sudden cardiac death from ischemia-induced arrhythmias or acute myocardial infarction.

In subjects using cocaine, individual myocytes may show "contraction" bands, which resemble those seen in pheochromocytoma-related myocardial disease consistent with early ischemic lesions of the myocardium. Established myocardial infarction may be observed in some cases.

Dysplastic disease and inflammatory arteritis

Fibromuscular dysplasia of coronary arteries

The usual observation of distinct layers in coronary arteries, intima, muscular media, and fibrous adventitia is altered in the case of dysplastic arteries. The media may have major deposits of connective tissue in the form of elastic fibers. The adventitia, which usually lacks elastic fibers, may have a proliferation of such fibers. In some cases the lumen

is narrowed [26–31] with the presenting symptom sometimes being sudden death.

Giant cell coronary arteritis

Giant cell coronary arteritis is characterized by leukocytic infiltration, including giant cells, in all layers of the arterial wall. This form of inflammatory arteritis may be restricted to the coronary arteries or may be part of a more generalized inflammatory state. Sudden death results from ischemia or infarction. This condition is distinct from the entity of giant cell myocarditis.

Acute arteritis of a coronary artery

Vasculitis of the coronary arteries may occur in different age groups. When vasculitis occurs in an infant or a child, it is most commonly due to mucocutaneous lymph node syndrome (Kawasaki disease). Acute lesions of the cardiac valves may also be seen [32]. Death in infancy or childhood is common. In cases where the acute lesions resolve, patients may develop multiple aneurysms of coronary arteries in later years. Sudden death may occur.

When acute arteritis occurs in adults, it most often related to periarteritis nodosa. The lesions may involve any of the arterial sites, including the coronary or renal arteries, or mesenteric vessels. Aneurysm formation is common.

Aneurysms adjacent to annuli of the aortic and/or mitral valves

Chesler and associates [33] reported on myocardial aneurysms subjacent to the aortic and/or mitral valves. These aneurysms result from a congenital defect at the valve annulus, rather than as a result of myocardial infarction. Submitral aneurysms occur only subjacent to the posterior leaflet. Whereas aortic sinus aneurysm may arise from any of the three aortic sinuses, subaortic aneurysms occur only under the intermediate portion of the left aortic sinus. In the absence of rupture, the clinical presentation of these aneurysms results from valvular insufficiency, compression of the left coronary artery, or disturbance of the conduction system. In a case reported by Smith and associates [34], a young man with a subaortic aneurysm of the left ventricle died suddenly secondary to rupture of the asymptomatic aneurysm into the pericardium.

Primary dissecting aneurysm of a coronary artery

Claudon and coworkers [35] reviewed 24 cases, including two observed by the authors, of primary dissecting aneurysm of a coronary artery. These patients are usually young adults, female more commonly than male. Among those with the condition many are in the early postpartum period. The essential lesion is rupture of the intima with the formation of an intimal hematoma. The clinical manifestations take the form of either sudden death or acute myocardial infarction. Surgical bypass procedure [36] or percutaneous intervention may remove the coronary arterial obstruction in the setting of acute myocardial infarction.

Calcified aortic sinotubular ridge

There may be lesions in the aortic wall, adjacent to the coronary artery ostia, which may encroach on the lumen of the artery, resulting in obstruction. These lesions may particularly affect the left main coronary ostium. Although some have assumed these lesions to be atherosclerotic in nature, they are typically fibrocalcific. Tveter and Edwards [37], who presented this entity, indicated that the lesion is more similar to the calcific lesions seen in the aged. Occlusion of coronary arteries by calcified embolic material may occur.

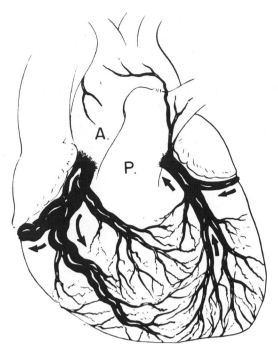

Figure 22 Origin of the left coronary artery from the pulmonary trunk.
Diagrammatic representation of the phenomenon of coronary blood supply coming partly from the pulmonary trunk.
The left coronary artery arises from the pulmonary trunk, while the right coronary artery is supplied by the aorta.

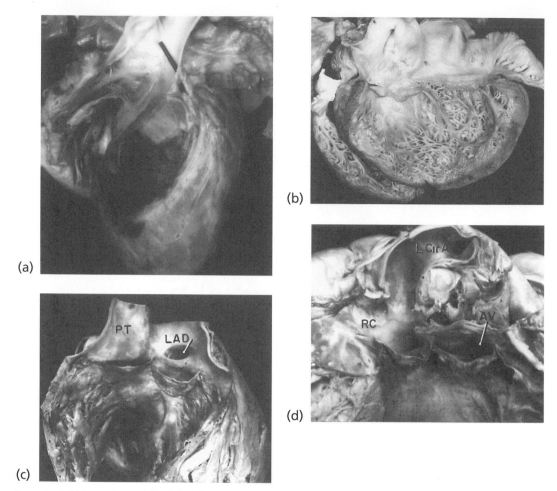

Figure 23 (a,b) Anomalous origin of the left coronary artery arising from the pulmonary trunk.
(a) Interior right ventricle and pulmonary artery. The probe is in the origin of the left coronary artery arising from the pulmonary trunk. The anomaly was responsible for death in infancy. (b) Left side of the heart in child with origin of left coronary artery from pulmonary trunk. The left ventricle is dilated, a frequent complication of this anomaly. Reprinted with permission from Noren et al. [19].
(c,d) Origin of left anterior descending coronary artery from the pulmonary trunk; left circumflex coronary artery arises from right coronary artery, which arises from the aorta.
(c) Right ventricle and pulmonary trunk (PT). Origin of left anterior descending (LAD) coronary artery is from pulmonary trunk. (d) Left circumflex coronary (L. Cir. A.) artery arose from the right coronary artery, which in turn arose from the aorta. Because of the high volume of blood through this functional left-to-right shunt there is aneurysmal dilatation of the vessels. The patient lived to 60 years.

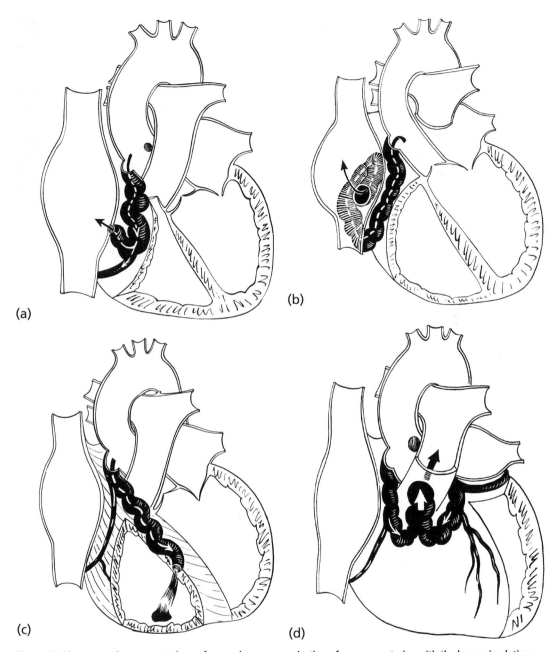

Figure 24 Diagrammatic representations of anomalous communication of coronary arteries with the lesser circulation.
(a) Right coronary artery communicates with right atrium. (b) Right coronary artery communicates with coronary sinus.
(c) Right coronary artery communicates with right ventricle. (d) Both coronary arteries arise from the aorta but also
communicate with the pulmonary trunk.

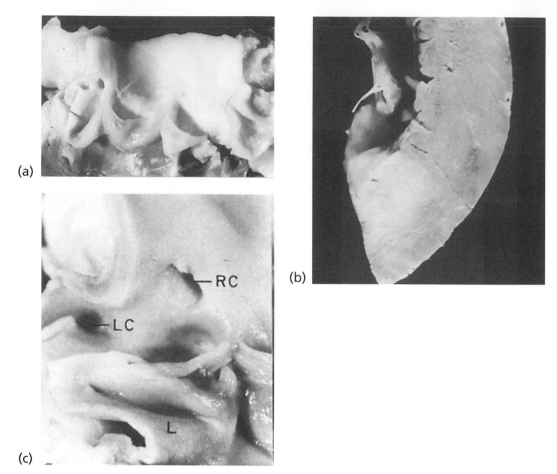

Figure 25 (a,b) Anomalous origin of coronary arteries from the same aortic sinus.
(a) Both coronary arteries arise from the right aortic sinus. Male, 8 years, who died following exercise. (b) Focus of left ventricular scar representing old myocardial infarction (same case as (a)).
(c) Origin of both coronary arteries from the left aortic sinus.
Both coronary arteries arise from the left aortic sinus, a phenomenon that may be associated with myocardial ischemia and sudden death.
Reprinted with permission from Mahowald et al. [21].

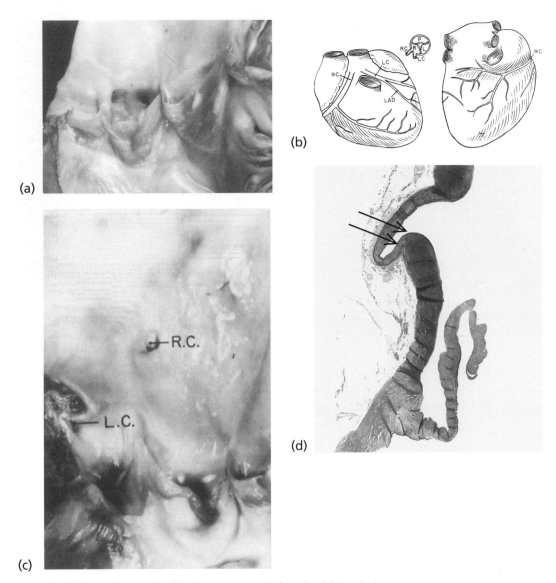

Figure 26 (a,b) Anomalous origin of both coronary arteries from the right aortic sinus.
(a) Both coronary arteries arise from the right aortic sinus. (b) Diagrammatic portrayal of both coronary arteries arising from the right aortic sinus as seen in the insert. The anterior view is less instructive than the cross-sectional insert. Reprinted with permission from Mahowald et al. [21].
(c,d) High origin of the right coronary artery.
(c) Anomalous high origin of right coronary artery. (d) Photomicrograph showing anomalous origin of right coronary artery (arrow) in a 7-year-old girl in whom sudden death occurred.

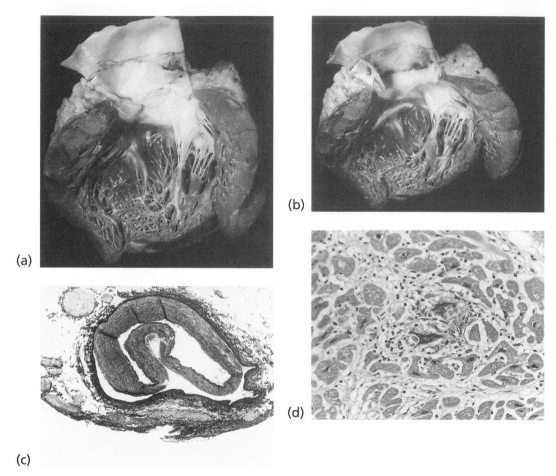

Figure 27 (a,b) Localized dissection of the ascending aorta causing acute obstruction to the origin of the left coronary artery.
(a) Left ventricle and the ascending aorta. Spontaneous tear of the ascending aorta. (b) The tear in the aorta has been reflected showing the site of origin of the left coronary artery.
(c) Catheter-related coronary artery complications.
Dissection of coronary artery during cardiac catheterization showing separation of the medial and partial compression of the true lumen by a false channel.
(d) Dissemination of talcum powder during cardiac catheterization.
Photomicrograph of myocardium showing particles of talcum powder with an associated inflammatory reaction with giant cell enveloping the talc. The talc presumably came from the gloves of the physician performing cardiac catheterization.

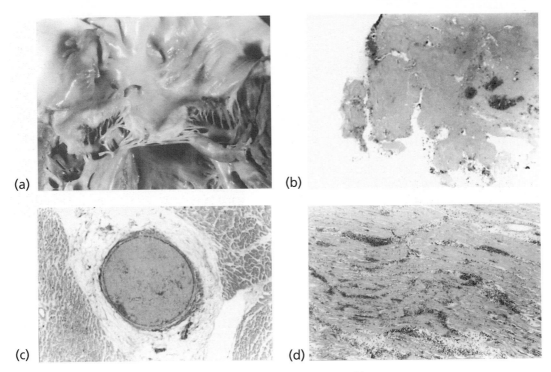

Figure 28 Coronary emboli caused by nonbacterial endocarditis in a 20-year-old woman.
(a) Mitral valve, vegetations of nonbacterial endocarditis. As is typical of nonbacterial endocarditis there is no evidence of valvular destruction. (b) Photomicrograph of embolus observed in a coronary artery. (c) Photomicrograph of coronary artery containing an embolus. (d) Photomicrograph of infarcted myocardium due to embolic nonbacterial vegetation.

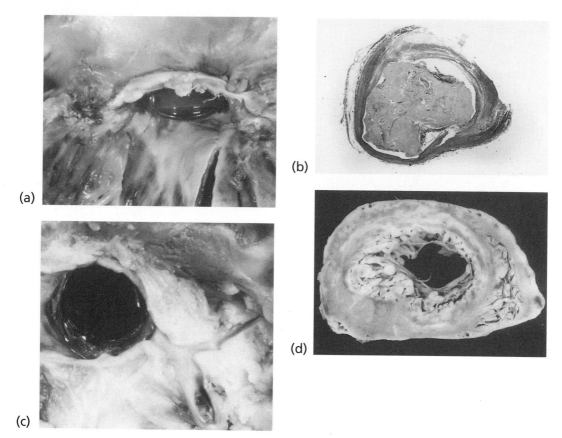

Figure 29 (a,b) Coronary embolus following mitral valve replacement in a 16-year-old girl.
(a) Mitral valve prosthesis. There are associated thrombosis and vegetations on the atrial surface of the prosthesis.
(b) A coronary artery containing an embolus.
Reprinted with permission from Ben-Shachar et al. [54]
(c,d) Postoperative aortic valve replacement with thrombosis and coronary embolism.
(c) Aortic valve replacement viewed from above with dissection revealing the left main coronary artery and its
bifurcation. There may be encroachment of the valve on the coronary ostium (arrow). (d) Acute myocardial infarction
resulting following aortic valve replacement. Male, 84 years.

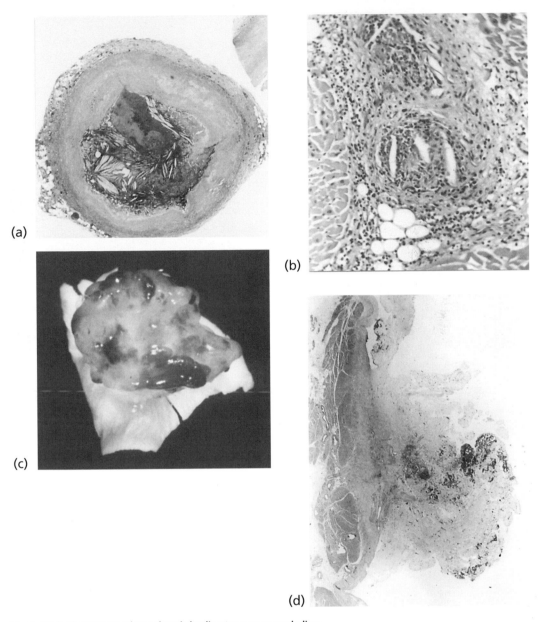

Figure 30 (a,b) Coronary atherosclerosis leading to coronary embolism.
(a) Coronary artery containing some atherosclerosis. Obstruction of the lumen by emboli composed of cholesterol crystals.
(b) Cholesterol crystals of coronary embolism in small vessels of myocardium.
(c,d) Left atrial myxoma as a source of coronary embolism.
(c) Surgical specimen of a left atrial myxoma. (d) Low power photomicrograph of tumor, a potential for embolism.

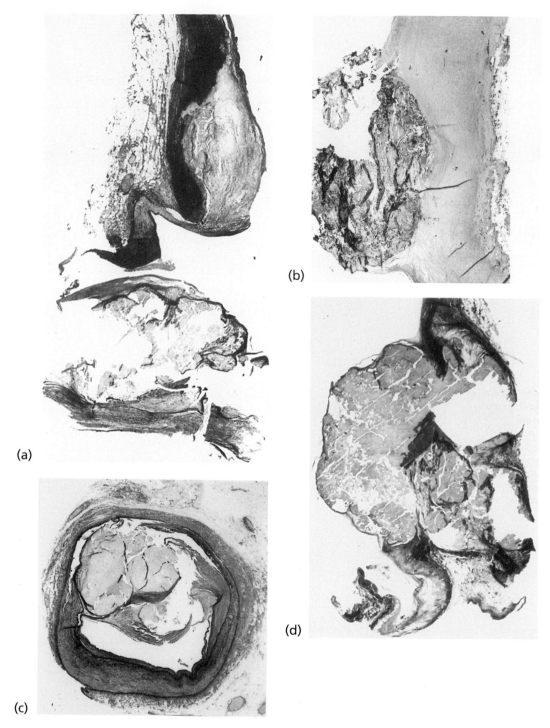

Figure 31 Nonatherosclerotic coronary arterial disease – calcified aortic sinotubular ridge.
(a) Photomicrograph. A coronary ostium is straddled by calcified lesions of aortic sinotubular ridge. (b) Aortic lesion represented by focus of calcification with the potential for embolization. (c) Coronary embolus of calcified material considered to be of aortic origin. (d) Wall of aortic sinus with amorphous calcified material that may contribute to a coronary embolism. Female, 76 years.
Reprinted with permission from Tveter and Edwards [37].

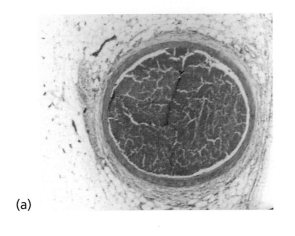

(a)

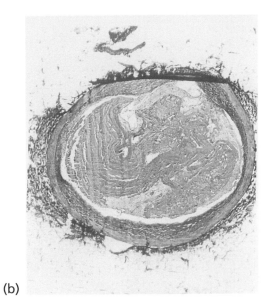

(b)

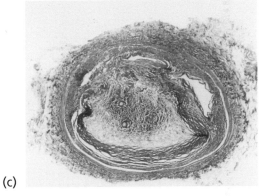

(c)

Figure 32 **Coronary embolism in three different patients involving large arteries in patients with mitral valvular disease.**
(a) Acute embolus of thrombotic material obstructing in the coronary artery resulting in acute myocardial infarction. (b) Early organization of an embolus.
(c) Organized embolus with associated atherosclerotic changes. Female, 53 years.
Reprinted with permission from Joassin and Edwards [159].

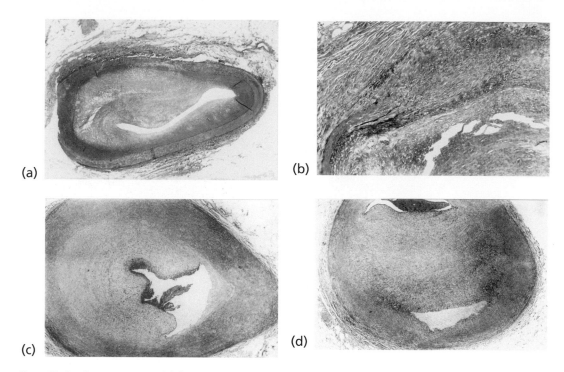

(a)

(b)

(c)

(d)

Figure 33 Cocaine coronary arterial disease.
(a,b) Elastosis of the walls associated with intimal fibrosis. The major intimal reaction with associated luminal narrowing is typical of chronic cocaine arteropathy. In some cases of cocaine-related deaths, there may be coronary spasm without associated structural changes. (c,d) Elastosis and intimal fibrosis from cocaine.
Illustrations courtesy of William D. Edwards.

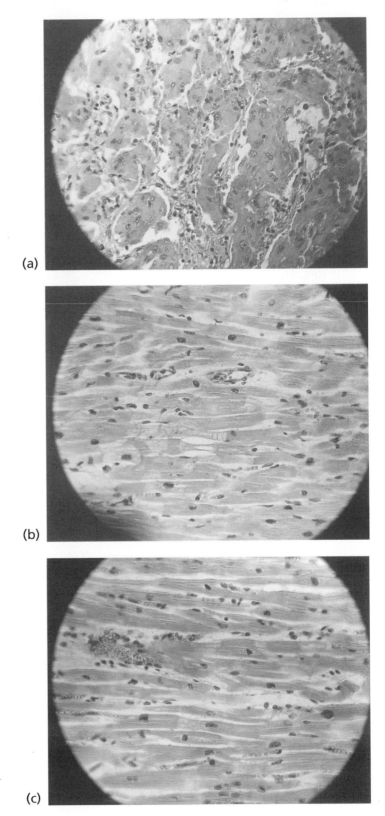

Figure 34 Myocardium in pheochromocytoma.
(a) Photomicrograph of adrenal pheochromocytoma. (b,c) Photomicrographs of myocardium showing "contraction bands" resulting from myocardial ischemia. Reprinted with permission from Edwards [177].

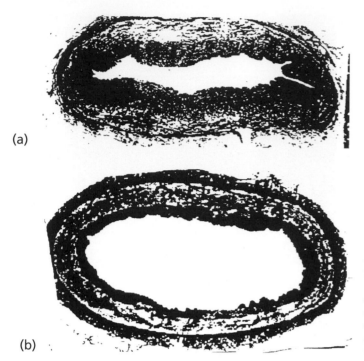

(a)

(b)

Figure 35 Dysplasia of coronary arteries causing sudden death. Male, 7 years.
(a) Malformation of histologic structures of coronary arteries characterized by abnormal formation of elastic tissue. (b) Media is the site of elastic fibers, which are abnormal in location.

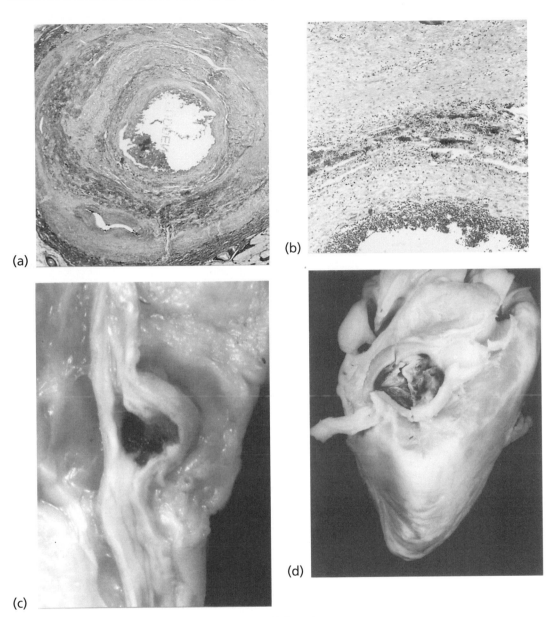

Figure 36 Mucocutaneous lymph node syndrome (Kawasaki disease).
(a) Coronary artery showing massive inflammatory response with luminal narrowing. (b) Each illustration shows an isolated aneurysm of a coronary artery. Although the clinical history for these cases is unavailable, the aneurysms have the appearance of Kawasaki disease.

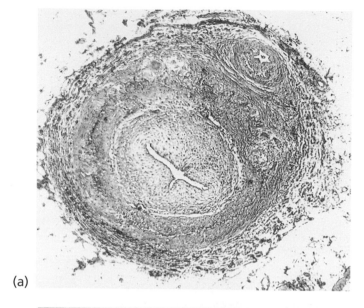

(a)

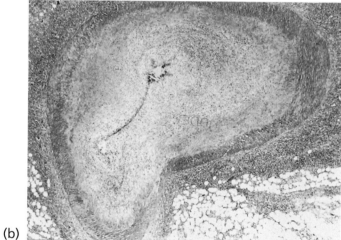

(b)

Figure 37 Giant cell arteritis of coronary arteries.
(a,b) Inflammatory response in all layers if the coronary artery including the adventitia. Giant cells are present. Female, 34 years.

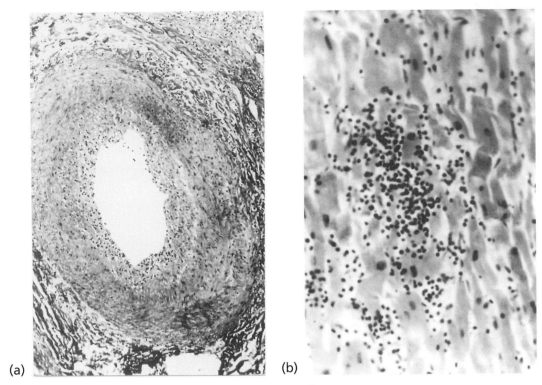

(a)
(b)

Figure 38 Post-transplant coronary vasculopathy with myocardial infiltrate.
Sudden death of a 16-year-old male following cardiac transplantation. (a) Postoperative major coronary vasculopathy following cardiac transplant. (b) Acute cellular infiltrate of the myocardium consistent with rejection.

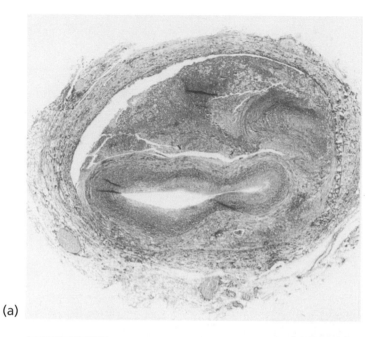

(a)

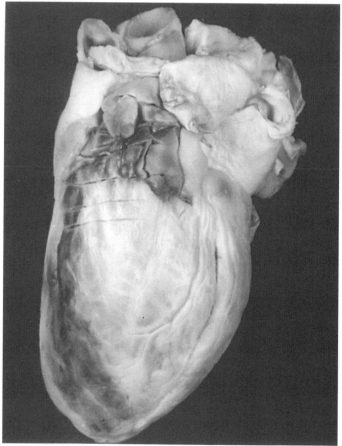

(b)

Figure 39 (a) Primary dissecting aneurysm of a coronary artery. Photomicrograph of left anterior descending coronary artery showing major intraluminal hematoma (dissection) that distorts and compresses the true lumen.
Reprinted with permission from Claudon et al. [35].
(b) Traumatic injury to epicardium and coronary arterial system. Discoloration of the epicardium corresponding to the course of the left anterior descending and the proximal portion of the left circumflex coronary artery. The discoloration represents subadventitial hemorrhage.

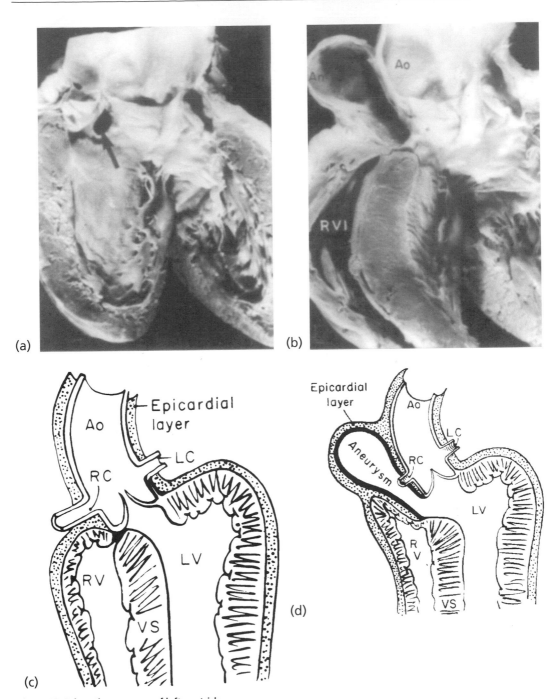

Figure 40 Subaortic aneurysm of left ventricle.
(a) The arrow points to the mouth of an aneurysm at the junction of the aorta and the left ventricular myocardium. Left ventricular blood escapes into the pericardial cavity through this defect. (b) A sagittal section through the ventricular septum, and the ostium of aneurysm shown at left, reveals that the aneurysm lies along the right side of the ascending aorta and superior to the right ventricular infundibulum. (c) Diagrammatic portrayal of the normal heart showing the relationship between the ostium of the aorta and the ventricular septum. (d) Hypothesis for separation of the aortic origin from the ventricular septum leading to a nonischemic aneurysm in the left ventricular base.
Reprinted with permission from Smith et al. [34].

CHAPTER 3

Myocardial disease

In this chapter we will consider various abnormalities of the myocardium that can result in sudden cardiac death. We have chosen to consider primary myocardial diseases associated with sudden death according to the following scheme:

(1) Dilated cardiomyopathy
(2) Restrictive cardiomyopathy
(3) Hypertrophic cardiomyopathy
  (a) Obstructive
  (b) Nonobstructive
(4) Right ventricular dysplasia
(5) Giant left atrial appendage
(6) Calcification of myocardium
(7) Myocarditis
(8) Chagas disease
(9) Alcohol-related cardiomyopathy

Dilated cardiomyopathy

Dilated cardiomyopathy has many causes. Cardiomegaly is the most prevalent pathologic finding; some of the largest hearts in our collection fall into this category. The patients may be young, and sudden death is not uncommon. Clinically, heart failure is usually the predominant symptom but, occasionally, sudden death may be the initial clinical presentation. Dilated cardiomyopathy is usually characterized by hypertrophy and dilatation of the ventricles; scarring and other forms of healing of inflammation vary. Some patients show extensive scarring; others do not.

The endocardium of the ventricles may be unusually thick in some patients with dilated cardiomyopathy. In cases of this type the diagnosis of endocardial fibroelastosis had been made as the primary cardiac condition. In recent years the classification of fibroelastosis has changed. Most people encountering fibroelastosis classify the disorder as secondary to a restrictive cardiomyopathy.

Severe mitral insufficiency is not uncommon in patients with dilated cardiomyopathy. Clinically, one has to determine whether the mitral insufficiency is primary or secondary to the underlying myopathy. With this approach, there are individuals who have been subjected to mitral valve repair or replacement on the basis of the theory that the mitral valve malfunction was the primary cause for disease.

Restrictive cardiomyopathy

Restrictive cardiomyopathy is one of the most intriguing phenomena among categories of heart disease. Basically, the ventricles resist dilatation and diastolic filling [38]. According to Fernando and associates [39], restrictive cardiomyopathy may be divided into several functional categories, which they designate as types A, B, and C. Type A is characterized by pulmonary and systemic venous congestion. The restrictive pattern is found in the inlet of both ventricles. The atria are large; the ventricles are small or normal. The differential diagnoses of the condition include constrictive pericarditis and systolic pump dysfunction. The type B condition is characterized by pulmonary venous congestion, pulmonary hypertension, and dilatation of the left atrium and right-sided chambers with a normal or small left ventricle. In the type C condition, there is restriction in the inlet of the right ventricle with a giant right atrium, systemic venous hypertension with low flow, and normal pressure in the pulmonary artery and left side of the heart. Some cases of restrictive cardiomyopathy have associated hypereosinophilic syndrome.

Hypertrophic cardiomyopathy

Significant hypertrophy of the ventricular myocardium and classically asymmetrical increased width of the ventricular septum are seen in hypertrophic cardiomyopathy. Some patients exhibit left ventricular outflow obstruction, while others have no obstruction. Hypertrophic cardiomyopathy may cause sudden death [40]. Many genetic mutations associated with hypertrophic cardiomyopathy have now been recognized, some of which have a relatively benign natural history, while other mutations carry a much higher risk of sudden death. In some cases the hypertophy may cause subaortic stenosis. If subaortic stenosis is present, the basis for obstruction may be the so-called systolic anterior motion of the mitral valve [41]: the mitral valve is not entirely closed during systole, and the anterior mitral leaflet and associated chordal structures are retained in a subaortic position. The anterior leaflet of the mitral valve impinges on the ventricular septum causing outflow track obstruction and some degree of mitral regurgitation. Sudden death occurs in these patients, particularly during exercise. The myocardium of the ventricular septum shows a peculiarity in structure known as "myocardial disarray" with prominent arteries.

In some cases of ventricular hypertrophy, care should be taken to distinguish obstructive hypertrophic cardiomyopathy from nonobstructive hypertrophic cardiomyopathy. Membranous subaortic stenosis, in contrast to hypertrophic cardiomyopathy, may be a primary disorder of the cardiac skeleton and may be associated with defects of the membranous ventricular septum. It is characterized by columns of collagen in the subaortic area of the outflow tract of the left ventricle and may lead to progressive outflow track obstruction and sudden death. Secondary ventricular hypertrophy in the body of the left ventricle may develop in patients with membranous subaortic stenosis, potentially leading to confusion of this entity with primary hypertrophic cardiomyopathy.

Right ventricular dysplasia

The entity of right ventricular dysplasia (also known as Uhl's anomaly) is characterized by loss of myocardium or fatty replacement of myocardium, particularly of the right ventricle [42]. This condition tends to occur more frequently in males, and some families have multiple affected members. While classically the condition involves only the right ventricle, there are cases in which the left ventricle is affected. In a report by Lee and associates [27], sudden death occurred in a patient with left ventricular fibrosis and fibromuscular dysplasia of the small intramyocardial coronary arteries. Congestive failure, arrhythmias, and sudden death are common.

Congenital aneurysm of giant left atrial appendage

Bramlet and Edwards [43] described a case of congenital aneurysm of the left atrial appendage. The case reported was that of a 55-year-old man who died of cerebral embolus originating from a thrombus in the left atrial appendage. Eleven years earlier, the cardiac silhouette on chest radiograph suggested a cardiac tumor or pericardial cyst. Fourteen published cases list the major manifestations of congenital aneurysm of the left atrial appendage as an abnormal cardiac silhouette in the x-ray, supraventricular tachycardia, and systemic embolization. Resection of the aneurysm is the recommended form of treatment.

Calcification of myocardium

Calcification of the myocardium may follow injury to the myocardium. Perhaps the most common cause of injury is prior myocardial infarction, but metabolic disorders may also result in ectopic calcification [44,45]. Sudden death has been observed in individuals with extensive myocardial calcification.

Myocarditis

Myocarditis is pathologically classified according to the "Dallas criteria," in which acute myocarditis is defined as "an inflammatory infiltrate of the myocardium with necrosis and/or degeneration of adjacent myocytes not typical of the ischemic damage associated with coronary artery disease." A host of conditions may be associated with myocarditis, including the postpartum state; various viral agents, such as Coxsackie B, CMV, and HIV; as well as chicken pox, measles, and poliomyelitis. Acute myocarditis seen in Lyme disease which results from infection with the spirochete *Borrelia burgdorferi*. The majority of cases of myocarditis are nonbacterial in origin. Classically, the condition is characterized by necrosis of myocardium with a cellular infiltrate. With time this leads to removal of myocardial fibers with secondary fibrosis and scarring of the myocardium. Pathologically myocarditis is frequently associated with corresponding pericarditis. Some cases of myocarditis display giant cells in the infiltrate. In some cases of acute myocarditis, the cellular infiltrate is heavily eosinophilic. Eosinophilic myocarditis is frequently a manifestation of drug-induced hypersensitivity. In chronic situations the cellular infiltrate may resolve and the myocardium is characterized by scarring with thickening of the endocardium. Such cases may sometimes be classified simply as dilated cardiomyopathy.

Cardiomyopathy accounts for an increasing proportion of reported postpartum-related deaths of myocardial origin. Some of these have evidence of active myocarditis, while in other cases there is no detectable histologic abnormality. The more than six-fold increased risk of death from cardiomyopathy among black women is larger than that for any other group. The increased reporting of these deaths might be due to improved case ascertainment [46].

Chagas disease

Chagas disease, common in South America, is said to be the most common cause of congestive heart failure worldwide. This condition results from the bite of the Reduviid bug, which transmits the infectious agent *Trypanosoma cruzi*. Acute infection is usually characterized by a self-limited febrile illness followed by a latent phase, which may last decades. The myocardium and the GI tract are most commonly affected in the chronic phase, often occurring 10–20 years following the initial infection. In this phase the organism is usually not present in the heart and the myocardial damage is probably mediated by an immune response. In the chronic state, heart failure and conduction disturbance are common. Sudden death may occur.

Alcohol-related cardiomyopathy

A complication of chronic alcohol ingestion may be its effect on the myocardium. There are probably several different mechanisms responsible for cardiac dysfunction among individuals who consume a large amount of alcohol. Metabolism of alcohol differs from individual to individual, and it has been speculated that some produce alcohol metabolites that are direct myocardial depressants. In others, chronic alcohol use may be associated with risk factors including nutritional deficiencies (thiamine) or chronic hypertension. The pathologic changes observed may include hypertrophy of the left ventricle and dilatation of the chambers. Morphologically it may be indistinguishable from idiopathic dilated cardiomyopathy. While hepatic disease may coexist, many patients with alcohol-related myopathy do not have evidence of hepatic cirrhosis. Patients with alcoholic cardiomyopathy may exhibit symptoms of congestive heart failure or may suffer from sudden arrhythmic death.

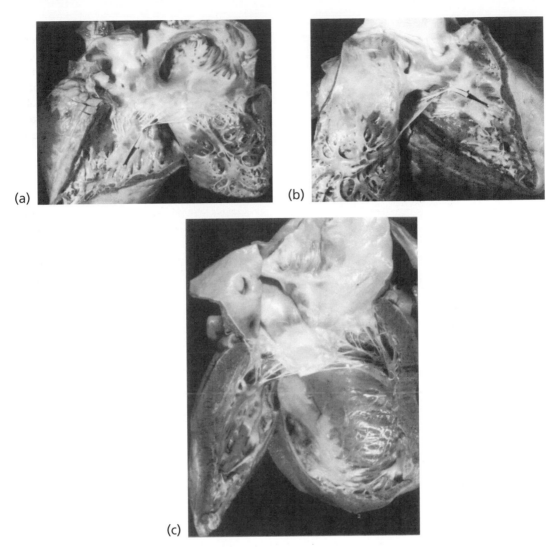

(a)

(b)

(c)

Figure 41 Dilated cardiomyopathy. Male, 35 years.
Dilated cardiomyopathy with marked cardiac hypertrophy. Cardiac weight 640 g. Diffuse endocardial fibrosis, normal coronary arteries. (a) Right atrium and right ventricle demonstrating marked endocardial thickening. (b) Right ventricle and pulmonary artery. Focal endocardial fibrosis within the right ventricle. (c) Left atrium and left ventricle. Marked chamber dilatation with endocardial fibrosis of the left ventricle. Mitral valve is normal.

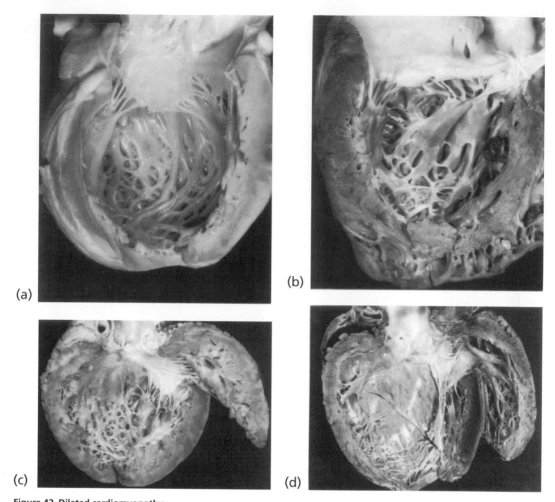

(a)

(b)

(c)

(d)

Figure 42 Dilated cardiomyopathy.
Illustrations of several cases. (a) Hypertrophy of the wall of the left ventricle with dilatation of the chamber. Male, 21 months. (b) Left ventricular hypertrophy in a patient with a dilated cardiomyopathy. Endocardial thickening. Female, 44 years. (c) Dilatation of left ventricle. Multiple sites of scarring of the myocardium. Heart weight 670 g. Female, 31 years. (d) Dilatation and scarring of the left ventricle. Male, 36 years.

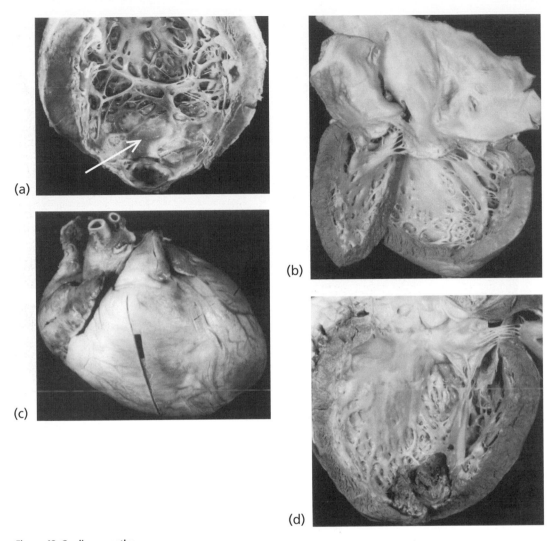

Figure 43 Cardiomyopathy.
(a) Left ventricular hypertrophy and dilatation with laminated thrombus at the cardiac apex (arrow). Cardiac weight 680 g. (b) Left side of heart with extensive scarring and aneurysmal dilatation of left ventricle. Dilatation of the left atrium. (c) External view of the heart. Major dilatation of left ventricle in a case of primary amyloidosis. The end-stage amyloid heart may have severe dilatation and can be confused with dilated cardiomyopathy. Male, 45 years. (d) Dilatation of left ventricle with thrombus at the apex. Male, 46 years.

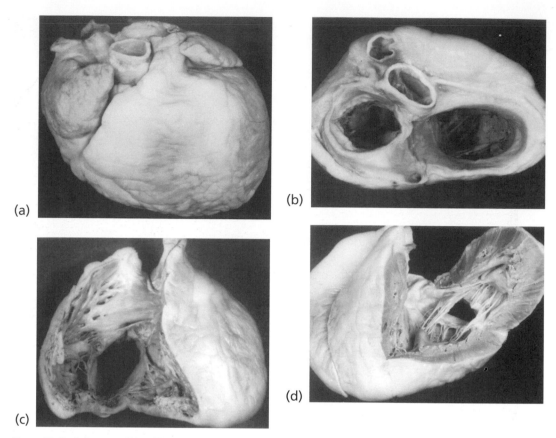

Figure 44 Healed myocarditis with cardiac dilatation and tricuspid insufficiency.
Male, 48 years. (a) Dilatation of right ventricle with prominence of the right atrial appendage. External view. (b) Base of the heart as viewed from above. Dilatation of mitral and tricuspid annuli. (c) Right ventricle dilatation. Internal view. (d) Left ventricle; mild hypertrophy of wall.

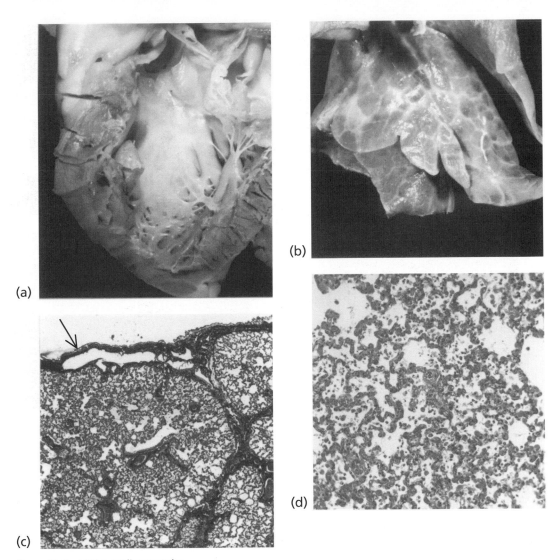

Figure 45 Restrictive cardiomyopathy.
Marked enlargement of left atrium and endocardial fibroelastosis within the left atrium and left ventricle. Right ventricular hypertrophy. Right atrial enlargement. Acute pulmonary venous hypertensive changes with dilatation of interlobular pulmonary lymphatics and veins. Female, 11 months. (a) Interior view of the left side of the heart. Endocardial fibroelastosis of atrium and ventricle. (b) Gross specimen. Pleural surface of lung. Focal congestion with prominent pleural lymphatics. (c) Lower power photomicrograph of lung showing a prominent lymphatic on the surface (arrow). This may be apparent on chest x-ray as Kerly B lines. (d) Pulmonary parenchyma showing alveolar congestion.

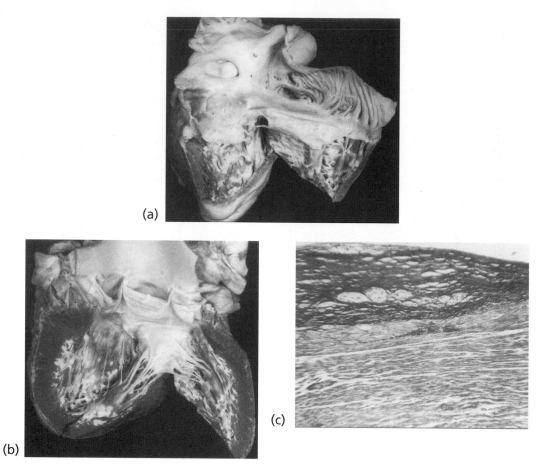

Figure 46 Metastatic adenocarcinoma in endocardium of both ventricles mimicking restrictive cardiomyopathy. Female, 52 years.
(a) Right side of heart. Interior right ventricle shows endocardial thickening from metastatic carcinoma in the endocardium. (b) Interior left ventricle showing metastatic carcinoma in the endocardium. (c) Photomicrograph of endocardium of right ventricle showing in the upper half of the image metastatic adenocarcinoma surrounded by well-established fibrous interstitium. The lower portion shows normal myocardium. This situation, sometimes referred to as *scirrhous carcinoma*, can lead to restrictive filling of one or both ventricles.
Reprinted with permission from Ocel et al. [107].

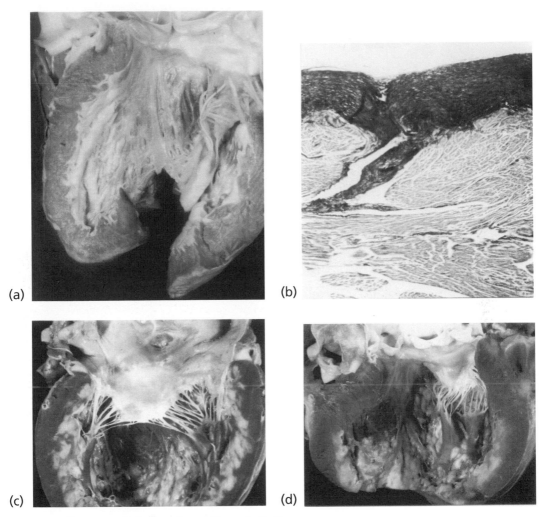

(a)

(b)

(c)

(d)

Figure 47 (a,b) Cardiomyopathy in patients with neoplastic disease.
Endocardial fibroelastosis resembling previous case, but without tumor. Female, 62 years. (a) Interior left ventricle
showing endocardial fibrosis in a patient with metastatic cancer, but without evidence of metastatic tumor.
(b) Photomicrograph of left ventricle including thickened endocardium. In spite of the fact that the patient had a
malignant tumor, the microscopic evaluation of the thickened endocardium reveals no tumor. This may represent a
paraneoplastic phenomenon.
(c,d) Myologic leukemic infiltration of the myocardium.
(c) Mitral valve and left ventricle. The nearly white leukemic infiltration is mostly subendocardial. (d) Left ventricle and
aorta demonstrating the leukemic infiltrate more prominent in the apical half of the ventricle. Male, 46 years.

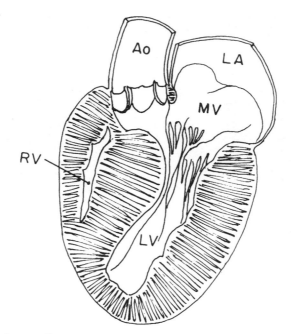

Figure 48 Hypertrophic cardiomyopathy.
Hypertrophic cardiomyopathy with left ventricular outflow track obstruction may mimic aortic stenosis or membranous subaortic stenosis. In classic hypertrophic cardiomyopathy, the ventricular septum is hypertrophied and contains an abnormal distribution of myocardial fibers, histologically referred to as *myocardial disarray*. The associated lesion of the anterior leaflet of the mitral valve is commonly called systolic anterior motion (SAM) of the mitral valve, and this phenomenon occurs throughout the cardiac cycle. The abnormal position of the mitral leaflet may be responsible for obstruction of the left ventricle outflow track and sudden death.
Muscular subaortic stenosis.
The ventricle septum is hypertrophied and the anterior leaflet of the mitral valve obstruct the outflow from the left ventricle.
Reprinted with permission from Maron et al. [40].

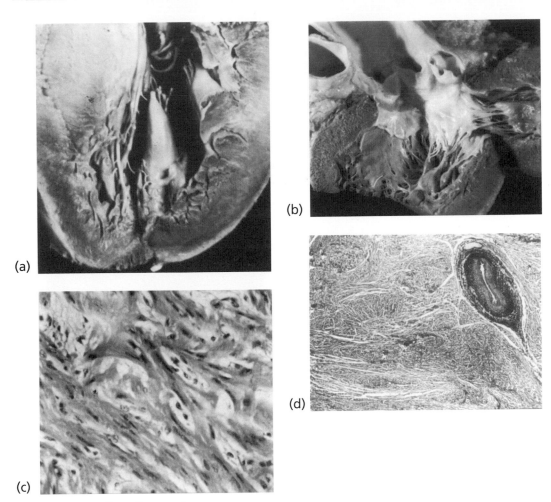

Figure 49 Hypertrophic cardiomyopathy.
(a) The left ventricle. Ventricular septum to the left. The septum is massively hypertrophied but the remaining portions of the left ventricle also demonstrate marked hypertrophy. (b) Outflow tract of left ventricle showing a fibrous patch on the ventricular septum caused by systolic anterior motion of the mitral valve. (c) Photomicrograph of ventricular septum showing classical disarray of the myocardial fibers. (d) Prominent intramyocardial artery in an area of classical disarray of the myocardial fibers.

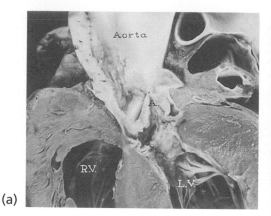

(a)

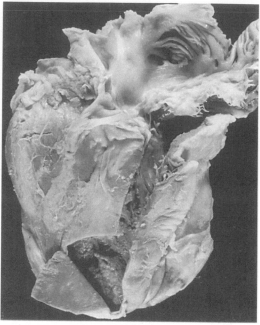

Figure 51 Right ventricular dysplasia.
Opened right ventricle shows the thinning of the right
ventricular wall in a case of right ventricular dysplasia (also
called Uhl's anomaly). Male, 72 years.

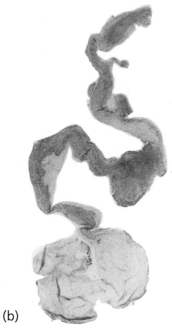

(b)

Figure 50 (a) Membranous subaortic stenosis.
View of the left ventricular outflow track and aorta. There
is a mural proliferation of fibrous tissue in the outflow
tract of the left ventricle that encroaches upon the aortic
valve. The fibrous tissue creates subaortic stenosis.
(b) Subaortic stenosis caused by a pedunculated fibroma.
A pedunculated lesion causing subaortic stenosis that was
relieved by resection.
Reprinted with permission from Gomes et al. [160].

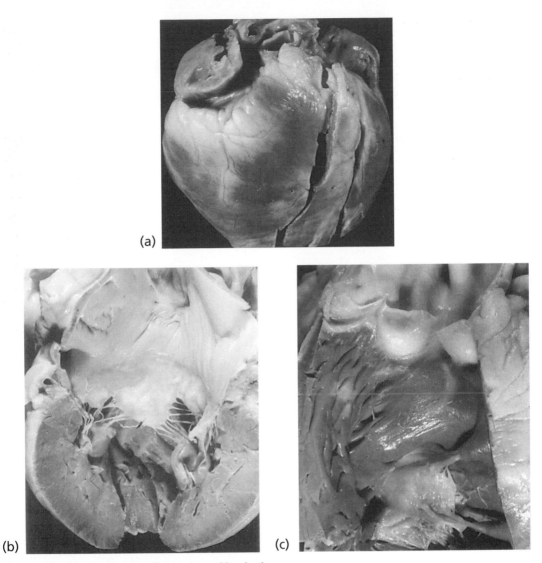

Figure 52 (a) Dilated cardiomyopathy causing sudden death.
External view of the heart of a 17-year-old boy who died suddenly. The right ventricle is prominent suggesting right ventricular hypertrophy and dilation. There was biventricular dilation.
(b,c) Nonobstructive hypertrophic cardiomyopathy causing sudden death.
Nonobstructive hypertrophic cardiomyopathy with symmetric left ventricular hypertrophy. Heart weight 765 g in a 48-year-old male. (b) Left side of heart. Major hypertrophy of the wall of the left ventricle. (c) Right ventricular outflow tract and pulmonary valve demonstrating major hypertrophy of the right ventricular muscle.

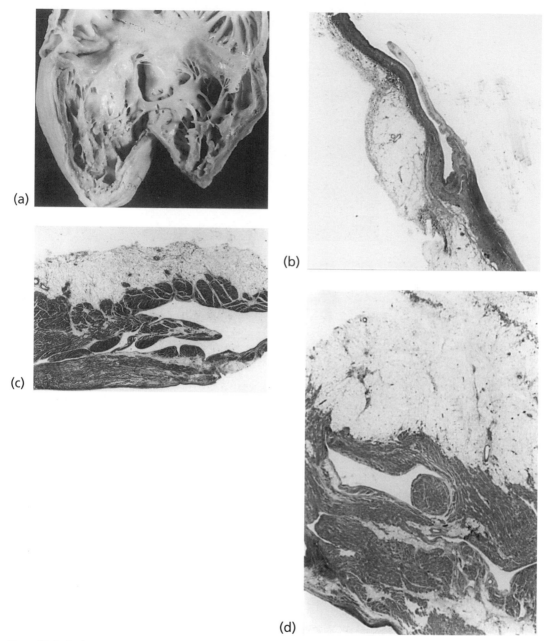

Figure 53 Arrhythmogenic right ventricular dysplasia causing sudden death.
Male, 35 years. (a) Interior of right ventricle showing enlargement of the cavity. (b) Low-power photomicrograph of a part of the right ventricle showing major replacement of the muscle by adipose tissue. (c,d) Two examples of excessive adipose tissue in epicardial portion of the right ventricle. The thin right ventricle may be particularly susceptible to rupture at the time of diagnostic right ventricular biopsy.

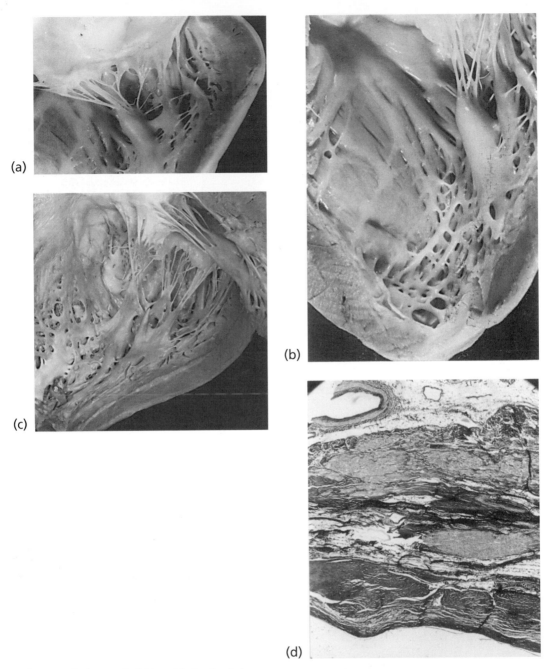

Figure 54 Arrhythmogenic right ventricular dysplasia.
(continued from previous case). (a,b) Two views of the left ventricle showing foci of replacement of myocardium by adipose tissue. Male, 35 years. (c) A portion of the left ventricle showing myocardial displacement by adipose tissue. (d) Photomicrograph of the left ventricle showing major replacement of myocardium by adipose tissue. Left ventricular lesion, as illustrated, may be seen in patients with classical right ventricular dysplasia. In this case, the dominant lesions were in the left ventricle.

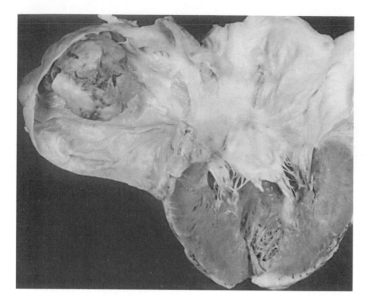

Figure 55 Congenital aneurysm of giant left atrial appendage.
Bramlet and Edwards described a case of congenital aneurysm of the left atrial appendage. The case reported was that of a 55-year-old man who died suddenly of a cerebral embolism originating in a thrombus in a congenital aneurysm of the left atrial appendage. Left side of heart: the left atrial appendage lies on the left and contains a mural thrombus. Left ventricular hypertrophy is also noted.
Reprinted with permission from Bramlet and Edwards [43].

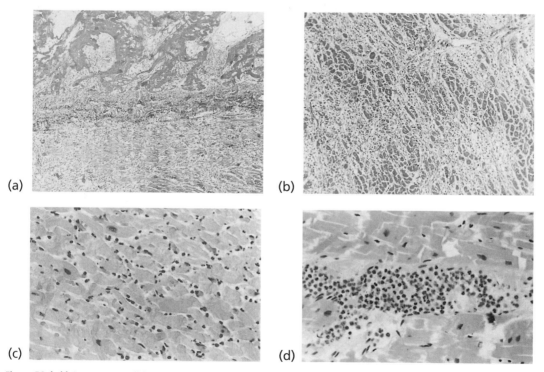

Figure 56 (a,b) Acute myocarditis.
(a) Photomicrograph of the visceral pericardium (upper half) and myocardium (lower half) showing pericarditis and myocarditis with an intense inflammatory infiltrate. (b) Acute myocarditis with cellular inflammatory infiltrate and myocyte necrosis.
(c,d) Acute myocarditis with sudden death.
(c) Leukocytes invade strips of myocardium. (d) Interstitial connective tissue infiltrated with lymphocytes with evidence of myocyte damage. Female, 18 years.

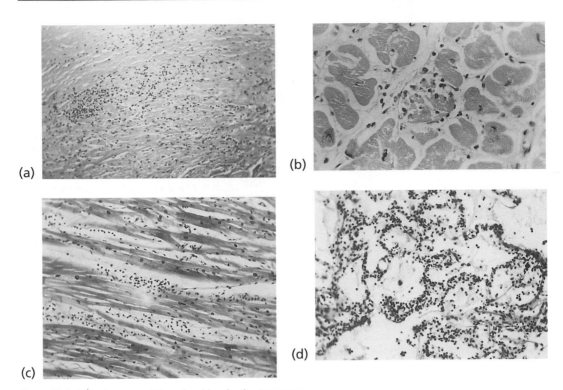

Figure 57 (a,b) Acute myocarditis and sudden death – two cases.
(a) Male, 6 years. About two weeks after recovery from chicken pox; the patient died suddenly. There is a heavy inflammatory infiltrate throughout the myocardium. (b) Acute myocarditis without identification of organism. One small zone of myocytes is undergoing phagocytosis by leukocytes. Female, 20 years.
(c,d) Early postpartum myocarditis.
(c) Acute interstitial myocarditis. (d) Early pneumonitis in a patient with acute postpartum myocarditis and sudden death.

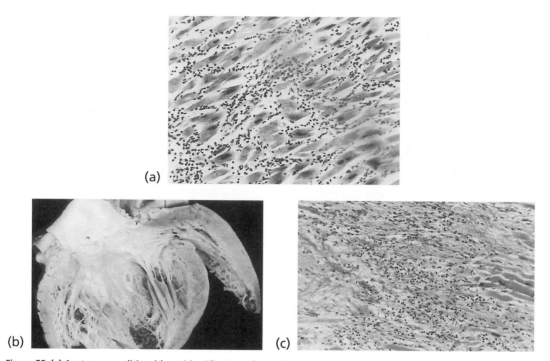

Figure 58 (a) Acute myocarditis without identification of organism.
Sudden death in a 43-year-old male. (a) Myocardium shows heavy interstitial infiltration with leukocytes. There is prominent interstitial edema.
(b,c) Chronic active myocarditis with mural thrombus in left ventricle.
Chronic active myocarditis led to congestive heart failure and sudden death. Female, 12 years. (b) Left ventricle with mural thrombus in the apex. (c) Interstitial leukocytic reaction between columns of myocardium. There is myocardial necrosis along with removal of myocytes.

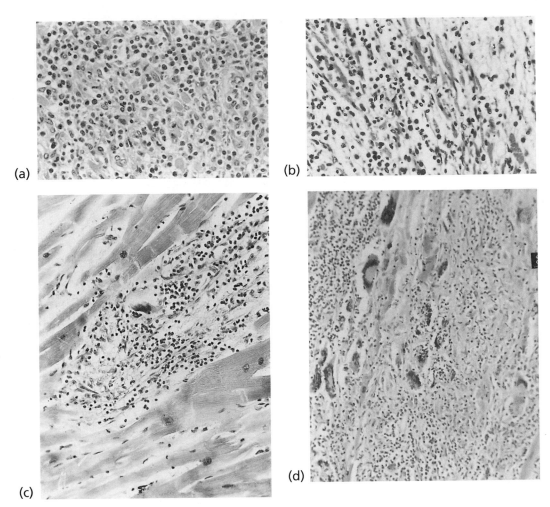

(a) (b) (c) (d)

Figure 59 (a,b) Fulminant diffuse transmural eosinophilic myocarditis.
(a) Lower power photomicrograph of the left ventricular myocardium demonstrating a heavy infiltration of leukocytes, predominantly eosinophils. There is extensive myocardial removal. (b) Photomicrograph of left ventricle. Along with the eosinophilic infiltrate, some remnants of necrotic myocytes can be identified.
(c,d) Giant cell myocarditis.
(c) Myocardium. Focus of giant cells and various leukocytes. (d) Myocardium with major leukocytic and giant cell infiltration. Sudden death is a common presentation for giant cell myocarditis.

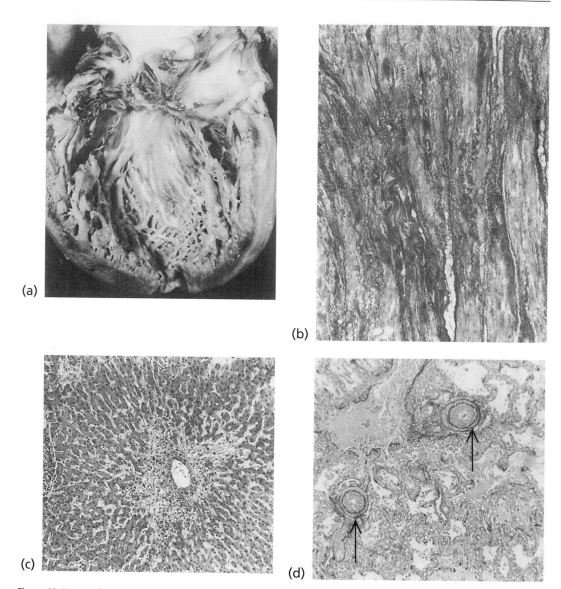

Figure 60 Remote history of myocarditis with extensive scarring of left ventricle and secondary mitral insufficiency.
Female, 25 years. (a) Left ventricle and left atrium. A mitral prosthesis was removed during the postmortem examination.
Endocardial fibroelastosis and dilation of left ventricle are present. (b) Photomicrograph of myocardium showing
extensive scarring of the myocardium. (c) Liver. Central vein with passage congestion "nutmeg liver." (d) Histology of lung
showing small arteries with occlusive intimal proliferation (arrows), presumably secondary to chronic elevation of
left-sided filling pressures.

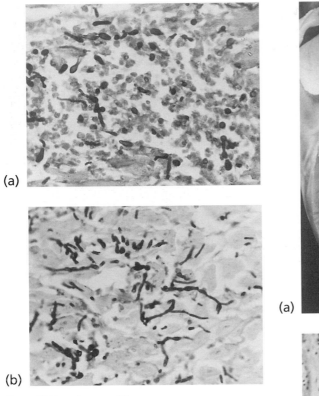

(a)

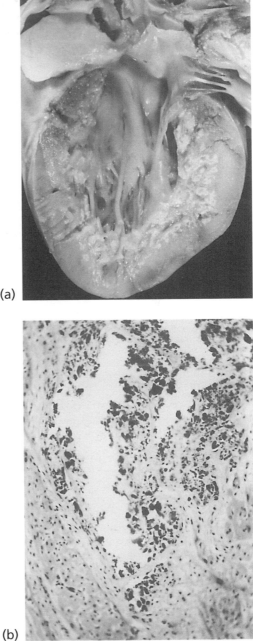

(a)

(b)

Figure 61 Fungal myocarditis.
(a) Photomicrograph of the left ventricle. Abscess of myocardium containing fungal organisms along with a cellular infiltrate. (b) Interstitial infiltration of myocardium by fungal organisms.

(b)

Figure 62 Calcification of myocardium in an infant.
(a) An infant suffered temporary cardiac arrest during surgery and died several weeks after the operation. The left ventricle shows areas of calcification as white discolorations. "Ischemic" (necrotic) areas of myocardium became quickly calcified. (b) Low power photomicrograph of myocardium. Dark stains indicate calcification of myocardial fibers.

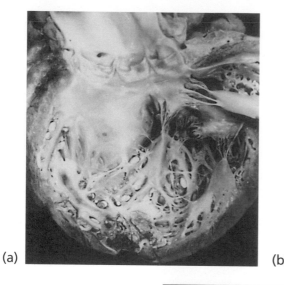

(a)

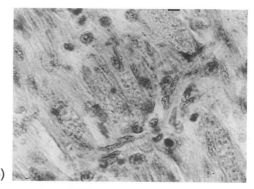

(b)

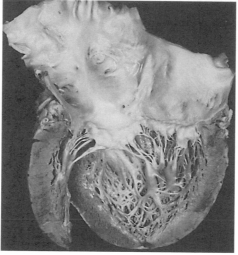

(c)

Figure 63 (a,b) Chagas myocarditis.
(a) Left ventricle in Chagas myocarditis. Ventricular dilatation and endocardial fibroelastosis. Apical mural thrombus.
(b) Photomicrograph of Chagas myocarditis showing *Trypanosoma cruzi* in myocardial fibers.
(c) Alcoholic myopathy. Male, 67 years.
Left side of heart. Dilatation of left atrium. Left ventricle is dilated to minor degree. The morphologic features are indistinguishable from idiopathic dilated cardiomyopathy. Sudden death without heart failure.

CHAPTER 4

Diseases of the Conduction System

Diseases of the conduction system are numerous and varied. The authors have selected a few representative entities for this section: complete heart block as a consequence of primary tumor of the atrioventricular node [47], complete heart block associated with aortic stenosis and surgical replacement of the aortic valve [48], and congenital complete heart block. Among women with lupus erythematosus who bear children, complete heart block is recognized in some of the offspring [49]. Congenital complete heart block, treated or untreated, in the infant may be followed by cardiac hypertrophy and its consequences.

Inflammatory diseases may involve the conduction system and cause complete heart block and other forms of delayed conduction. Chagas disease (chapter 3) is probably the leading cause of conduction disease on a global basis.

Dysplasia of the atrioventricular node may be seen as a cause of sudden death. Accessory pathways may lead to accelerated conduction and tachyarrhythmias. While Wolff-Parkinson-White syndrome may be the classic example of an accessory pathway, other types exist. The authors have observed a case of sudden death in a young woman because of the presence of a bundle of smooth muscle in the anterior leaflet of the mitral valve, presumably causing an accessory pathway.

The pathologic examination may reveal the underlying abnormality causing conduction disease, and the consequences of treating this disease with devices and drugs may also be observed. Chronic indwelling pacemaker and defibrillator leads may exhibit their own iatrogenic complication, including thrombus formation and valve dysfunction, and serve as a nidus for infection.

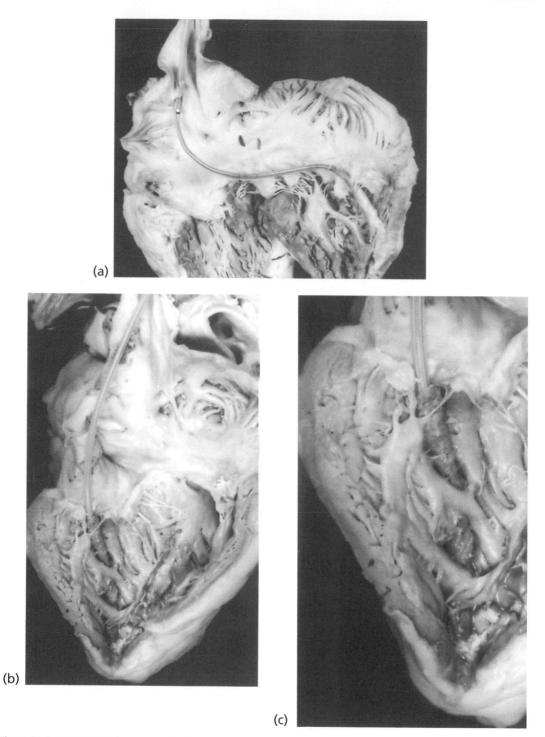

(a)

(b)

(c)

Figure 64 Consequences of pacemaker leads.
Illustrations from cases in which intravenous pacemaker leads have been in place for many months. (a) Right atrium and superior vena cava. The electrode lies attached to two sites: one at the superior vena cava–right atrium junction, the other adherent to the tricuspid valve. This may lead to tricuspid insufficiency. Male, 79 years. (b,c) The pacemaker electrode running from the superior vena cava through the right atrium to the right ventricle. Two views of the lead being surrounded by reactive connective tissue. Male, 72 years.
Reprinted with permission from Becker et al. [91].

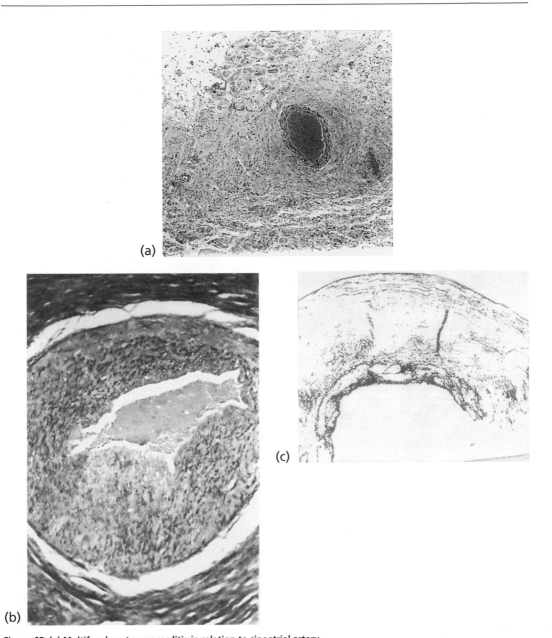

Figure 65 (a) Multifocal acute myocarditis in relation to sinoatrial artery.
(a) Photomicrograph showing a focus of acute inflammation adjacent to the sinus node artery, in a young woman with sudden death. This was the only pathologic abnormality found. Female, 29 years.
(b,c) Miscellaneous lesion of conduction system.
(b) Cellular proliferation (arterial dysplasia) in artery of sinus node. Sinus node ischemia may be responsible for sudden cardiac death. (c) Anterior mitral leaflet showing a column of smooth muscle running through the ventricular mitral side of the anterior leaflet; from a young woman who died suddenly. This may be the site of an accessory pathway for conduction ventricular.

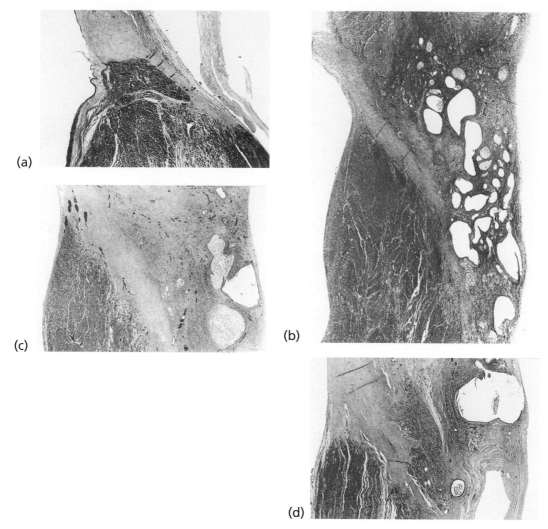

Figure 66 Mesothelioma of atrioventricular node causing sudden death.
(a) Atrioventricular node and surrounding right atrium and right ventricle. In this microscopic section no tumor is apparent. (b) Deeper cuts of the atrioventricular (AV) node. There are epithelial lined lystic spaces in the AV node representing a mesothelioma. (c,d) Details of the tumor. The mesothelioma is a benign cardiac tumor but may be responsible for sudden death. Premortem diagnosis is difficult.
Reprinted with permission from Ibarra-Perez et al. [47].

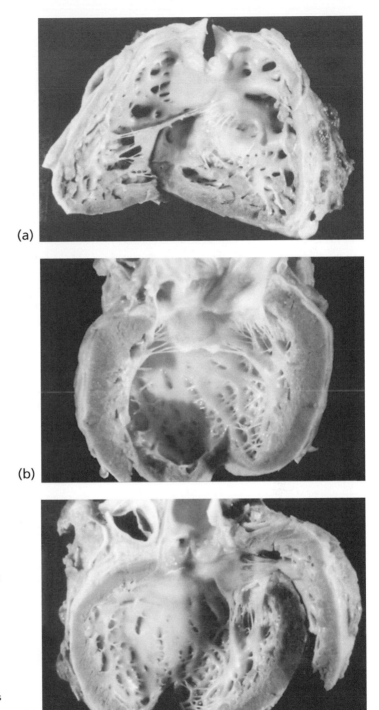

(a)

(b)

(c)

Figure 67 Congenital heart block.
Two-year-old male with congenital heart block, who was treated with a pacemaker. Despite treatment sudden death occurred. Examination of the heart revealed each chamber to be dilated.
(a) Right ventricle increased in volume with myocardial hypertrophy. (b) Left ventricle and left atrium. Dilatation of chambers with endocardial fibroelastosis.
(c) Left ventricle and aorta. Left ventricle is dilated. Dilation develops presumably because of increased diastolic filling time.

5 | CHAPTER 5

Systemic hypertension

One of the primary pathologic consequences of chronic hypertension, either primary or secondary type, includes the development of hypertrophy of the left ventricle [50,51]. Secondary hypertension is seen among patients with conditions that may include (1) renal arterial stenosis, (2) primary parenchymal disease of the kidney, (3) congenital obstruction of the urinary tract, (4) adrenal tumors or hyperplasias, and (5) coarctation of the aorta. Along with the development of hypertrophy, classically there occurs dilatation of the left ventricle. The left ventricle is enlarged and shows movement of the papillary muscles away from each other. The primary gross pathologic change resulting from hypertension is thickening of the myocardium and enlargement of the left ventricular chamber. Variations occur when the right ventricle is also hypertrophied and the left ventricle is infarcted because of coronary atherosclerosis. In patients with hypertension the small arteries and arterioles show an increase in the thickness of the medial layer. The intima may also show a major increase in cellularity leading to a pinpoint narrowing of the lumen. Regardless of the cause of the hypertension, complications of hypertension are the same. Recognized complications include atherosclerosis with its multiple manifestations. Other complications include left ventricular hypertrophy with restrictive ventricular filling, diastolic dysfunction, and pulmonary congestion.

Arteriosclerotic aneurysms of the abdominal aorta, as well as aortic dissection, are observed in patients with chronic hypertension.

In the patient with hypertension, the brain and cerebrovascular system are subject to a variety of complications, including cerebral infarction. Some are associated with cerebral thrombosis. In extensive infarction of the cerebrum, hemorrhage may occur in the brainstem. In some instances, the major cerebral complication is a ruptured aneurysm of the circle of Willis. The aneurysm may be of atherosclerotic basis or the so-called congenital aneurysm. Both of these aneurysms may develop or expand secondary to the hypertension. Aneurysms of the circle of Willis may be solitary or multiple. If the aneurysm is solitary and results in hemorrhage, it tends to involve the pia-arachnoid. In those cases in which survival occurs beyond the rupture of an aneurysm, a secondary rupture tends to hemorrhage into the cerebrum.

Regarding the "congenital" cerebral (berry) aneurysms, the wall of the aneurysm classically does not contain a medial layer; rupture, without warning, can lead to sudden death.

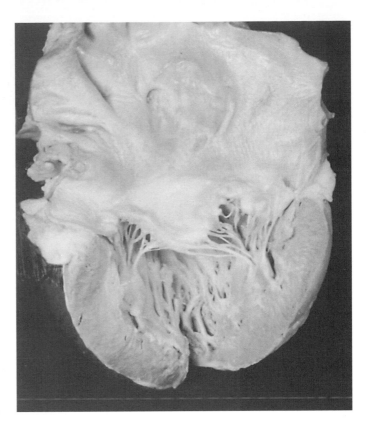

Figure 68 Cardiac effects of systemic hypertension.
Left side of heart in hypertension. Enlargement of left atrium and hypertrophy of the left ventricular wall.

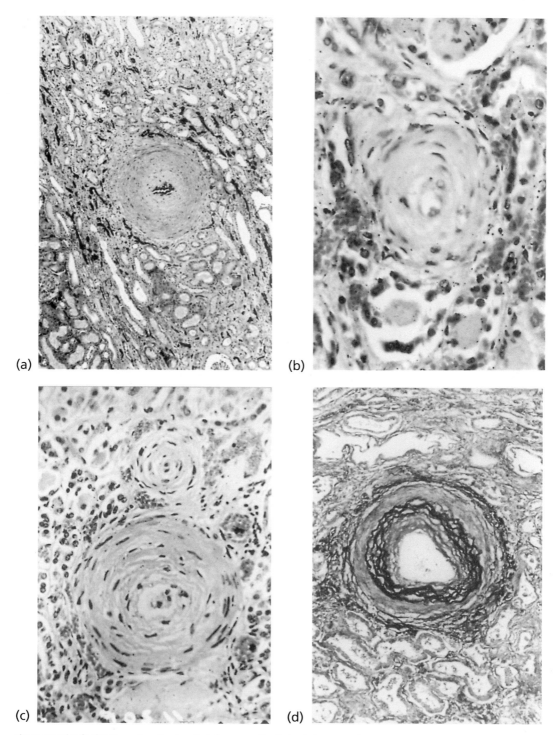

Figure 69 Histologic views of systemic arterioles or small arteries in hypertension.
(a,b) Small arteries in the kidney show prominent intimal proliferation. (c) Major intimal proliferation in a small artery showing the classic "onion peel" appearance consistent with malignant hypertension. (d) Small artery in the kidney shows early medial hypertrophy and intimal proliferation. The dark staining elastic tissue is prominently seen in the intima. Reprinted with permission from Lynch and Edwards [51].

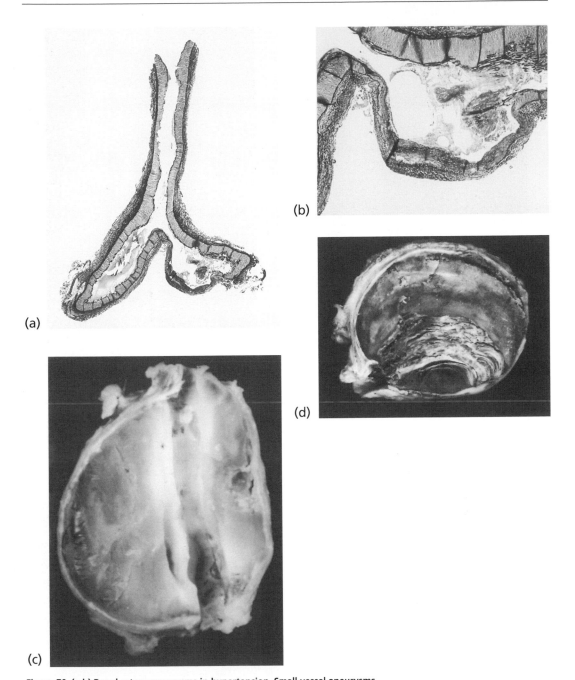

Figure 70 (a,b) Renal artery aneurysms in hypertension. Small vessel aneurysms.
(a) Low-power photomicrograph showing a renal artery with aneurysm in a branch. (b) Close-up view of the renal artery aneurysm shown in (a).
Reprinted with permission from Lynch and Edwards [51].
(c,d) Aneurysms of the main renal artery.
(c) Renal artery. Congenital aneurysm with thrombus. Male, 55 years. (d) Renal artery. Large aneurysm with associated thrombus.

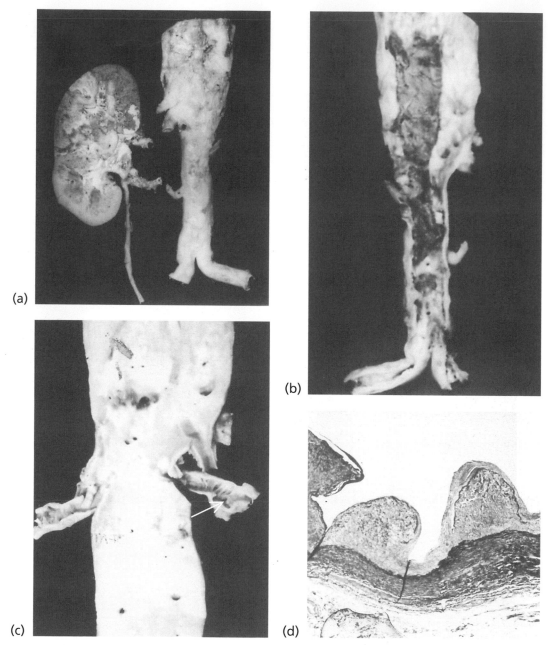

Figure 71 (a,b) Arterial obstruction to the kidney as a basis for hypertension.
Severe atherosclerosis with in situ thrombosis of abdominal aorta.
(a) Aorta and left kidney; infarction of kidney secondary to obstruction of the renal artery. (b) Interior of aorta showing extensive atherosclerosis, with aortic obstruction by thrombus.
Reprinted with permission from Lynch and Edwards [51].
(c,d) Fibromuscular dysplasia of renal arteries causing systemic hypertension.
(c) Renal arteries have been opened showing the corkscrew distribution of intimal lesions (arrows) causing luminal obstruction. (d) The cross section of renal artery shows the regular foci of proliferation, which collectively cause high degrees of luminal obstruction. The angiographic appearance of these areas of focal proliferation is referred to as the "string of beads" sign.

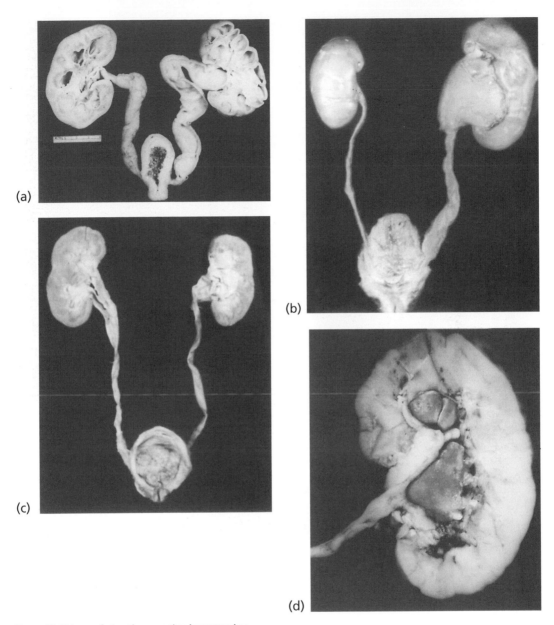

Figure 72 Urinary obstructions causing hypertension.
(a) Bilateral congenital hydroureter causing renal failure electrolyte abnormalities and hypertension. Male, 14 months sudden death. (b) Unilateral congenital hydroureter. (c) Carcinoma of bladder with bilateral hydroureter resulting in secondary hypertension. (d) Multiple renal calculi.

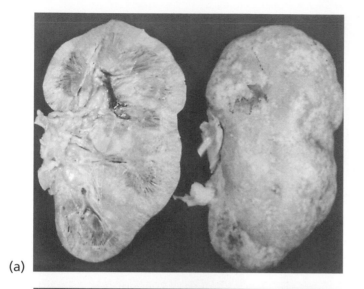

(a)

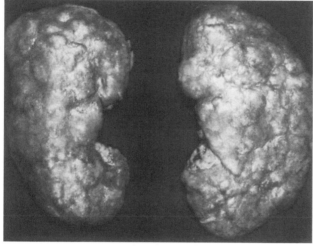

(b)

Figure 73 Acute and chronic pyelonephritis.
(a) Cut surface and exterior view of kidney in acute pyelonephritis.
(b) External surfaces of the kidneys in chronic pyelonephritis. Pyelonephritis leading to chronic hypertension and renal failure produce the substraight for sudden death.
Reprinted with permission from Lynch and Edwards [51].

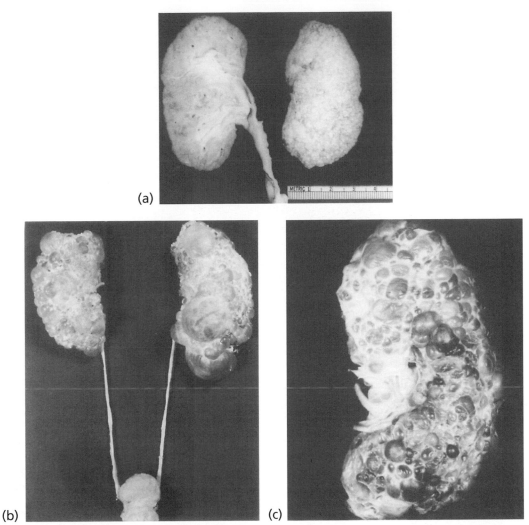

Figure 74 Systemic hypertension: Renal causes.
Diseases of the kidneys. (a) Chronic glomerulonephritis. (b) Both kidneys and ureters with bladder. A case of classical congenital polycystic kidneys. Male, 59 years. (c) Cut surface of a kidney in classical congenital polycystic kidney disease. Multiplicity of cysts replacing recognizable renal structure. Polycystic kidney disease may be associated with aneurysms of the circle of Willis, bicuspid aortic valve, and dilated cardiomyopathy.
Reprinted with permission from Lynch and Edwards [51].

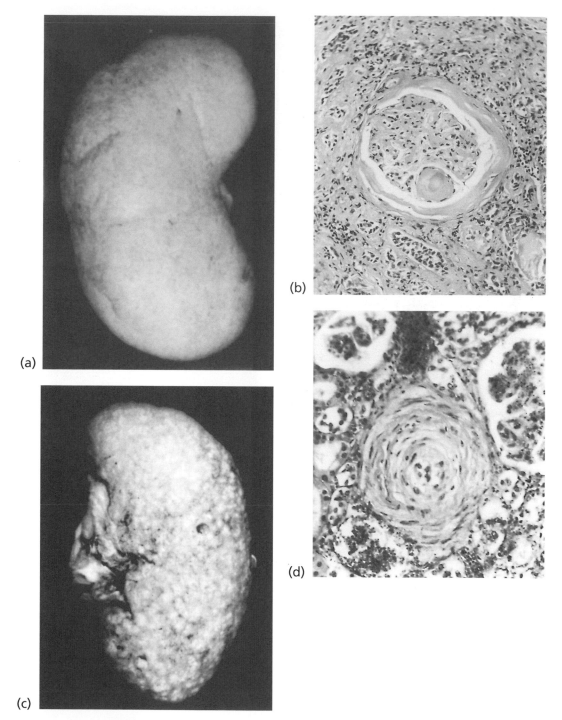

Figure 75 Systemic conditions.
Kidney with Kimmelstiel-Wilson disease secondary to diabetes. (a) External view of kidney showing a pale translucent appearance. Male, 33 years. (b) Photomicrograph. Nodular glomerulosclerosis resulting in hypertension and sudden death. Female, 70 years. (c) Scleroderma kidney, with cortical nodularity. Gross specimen of kidney.
(d) Photomicrograph of kidney with scleroderma showing major intimal proliferation as a cause of hypertension.
Reprinted with permission from Lynch and Edwards [51].

(a)

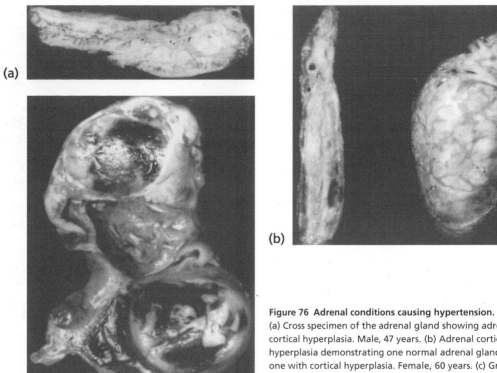

(b)

(c)

Figure 76 Adrenal conditions causing hypertension.
(a) Cross specimen of the adrenal gland showing adrenal cortical hyperplasia. Male, 47 years. (b) Adrenal cortical hyperplasia demonstrating one normal adrenal gland and one with cortical hyperplasia. Female, 60 years. (c) Gross specimen of an adrenal pheochromocytoma.
Reprinted with permission from Lynch and Edwards [51].

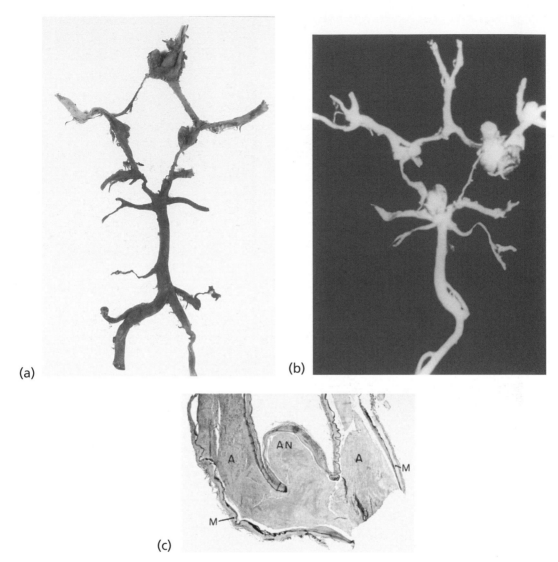

(a)

(b)

(c)

Figure 77 Cerebrovascular complications of hypertension causing sudden death.
(a,b) Two examples of patients with chronic hypertension and multiple berry aneurysms of the circle of Willis. (c) Photomicrograph of a portion of the circle of Willis with a berry aneurysm. AN-berry aneurysm; A-artery; M-arterial media. The wall of the aneurysm contains no medial layer.

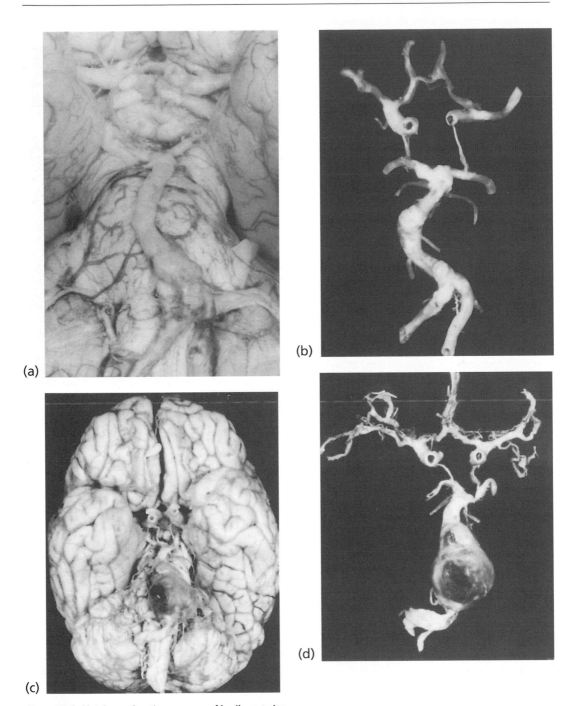

Figure 78 (a,b) Atherosclerotic aneurysm of basilar arteries.
(a,b) In two hypertensive patients the basilar arteries are involved with atherosclerosis. The course of the artery becomes tortuous. Male, 72 years.
(c,d) Brain and circle of Willis in a hypertensive patient with a basilar artery arteriosclerotic aneurysm that ruptured causing sudden death.
(c) Base of brain with meningeal hemorrhage in a 63-year-old man. (d) The basilar arterial aneurysm (arrow) has ruptured.

CHAPTER 6

Valvular heart disease

In this chapter, valvular disease as a cause of sudden death will be reviewed. The following selected topics will be presented: rheumatic heart disease affecting the mitral valve, causing either stenotic or regurgitant lesions; myxomatous mitral valve and other forms of mitral regurgitation, including papillary muscle dysfunction; calcification of the mitral ring; tricuspid regurgitation; aortic stenosis; aortic regurgitation; pulmonary valvular stenosis; and, infectious endocarditis. This chapter will also illustrate conditions that in some ways mimic infectious endocarditis, including nonbacterial endocarditis, lesions related to insertion of catheters, and atheromatous (cholesterol) embolism.

Some indication of the variety of valvular heart disease can be assumed from the surgical procedures done on cardiac valves. In a study that predated common mitral valve repair, Hanson and associates [52] studied 100 consecutive surgically excised mitral valves followed by insertion of prosthetic valves. The valves were classified according to primary conditions that resulted in their malfunction.

Rheumatic mitral valve disease (stenosis and/or insufficiency) accounted for 54% of the cases. Myxomatous changes (prolapse of the mitral valve) were present in 32 cases, among which 59% (19 cases) also had chordal rupture. Four of the cases had papillary muscle rupture and in seven cases papillary muscle dysfunction was the primary disorder. In one case infectious endocarditis was observed on a previously normal valve. In another case the pathology of valvular changes was indeterminate. Lupus erythematosus was diagnosed in one patient with mitral insufficiency. Mitral valve disease may present with chronic heart failure, arrhythmias, or sudden death.

Rheumatic heart disease

Rheumatic heart disease, while declining in the Western world, remains a major problem in underdeveloped or developing countries. In this section, the various changes in the valves observed are described. Rheumatic valvular disease stems from acute recurrent rheumatic fever. Rheumatic fever affects joints of the body and each layer of the heart. A famous pathologist of the last century was frequently quoted as saying, "Rheumatic fever licks the joints and bites the heart."

The specific histologic reaction of rheumatic inflammation in the heart is the Aschoff body. The Aschoff body is found in the endocardium, myocardium, and pericardium, while the inflammatory changes observed in the valve may be nonspecific. The reaction to the Aschoff body leads to fibrosis and the possibility of valvular calcification. As they affect the valves, these processes lead to stenosis, regurgitation, or both conditions at once [53]. Any of the valves of the heart may be affected but, as a practical matter, the valves of the left side of the heart are affected more commonly than the valves of the right side, and rarely, if ever, do you see right-sided involvement in the absence of left-sided involvement.

When the mitral or tricuspid valve is affected by rheumatic stenosis, there is classically a reduction in the caliber of the orifice, with fusion and fibrosis of chordae and calcification at the commissures. As the mitral valve becomes stenotic, the pressure in the left atrium and the pulmonary venous system becomes elevated. This results in dilatation of the left atrium; while the left ventricle is unaffected. There is a great tendency for thrombosis either in the atrial appendage or in the body of the left atrium [54]; it is especially common in patients with atrial fibrillation. The thrombi in the left atrium may occupy the orifice of the entering pulmonary veins. Rarely, a thrombus originating in the left atrium becomes trapped in the stenotic mitral valve. In hearts with mitral stenosis it is common to find effects of rheumatic fever on other valves [55,56]. As a consequence of elevated left atrial pressure, the dilated left atrium may displace the left main stem bronchus, which may in turn compress an adjacent pulmonary arterial segment. Mitral stenosis may result in hoarseness due to compression of the left recurrent laryngeal nerve because of elevation of the left bronchus and pulmonary artery. In patients undergoing mitral valve replacement, we have observed isolated cases with a laceration of the related myocardium. This may result in massive hemorrhage; however, in other cases the hemorrhage is contained leaving a false aneurysm at the site of the injury.

Mitral stenosis can result in pulmonary venous obstruction or elevated pressure within the pulmonary veins. Lesions within the pulmonary veins, such as those seen with intraluminal tumors, can mimic mitral stenosis. Pulmonary veno-occlusive disease may also have a similar presentation.

Mitral regurgitation

Mitral regurgitation allows blood from the left ventricle to flow into the left atrium with each systole. There are diverse causes of this disorder. The principal causes for the mechanism of mitral regurgitation are as follows:

1 Rheumatic heart disease
2 Myxomatous valvular disease
3 Papillary muscle dysfunction
4 Infectious endocarditis
5 Left ventricular failure
6 Rupture of the chordae, complicating either infectious endocarditis or myxomatous mitral valvular disease.

In rheumatic heart disease it is common that some degree of stenosis and regurgitation occur together, particularly affecting the mitral valve.

Rheumatic mitral regurgitation

There are three major anatomic manifestations of rheumatic mitral regurgitation:

1 Short leaflets without major fusion of the commissures
2 Fusion at one commissure, creating the "tear drop" form of mitral regurgitation
3 Fusion at both commissures, creating the "wedding ring" type of mitral regurgitation.

The theme "Mitral regurgitation begets mitral regurgitation" is illustrated. In mitral regurgitation of rheumatic origin, the posterior leaflet is displaced beyond the posterior position of the ventricle. This phenomenon tends to immobilize the affected leaflet and create further mitral regurgitation.

Myxomatous mitral valve

Many names are given to this condition: "floppy mitral valve," "myxomatous degeneration of the mitral valve," "ballooning mitral valve," "the redundant cusps syndrome," "mitral valve prolapse," and "systolic click murmur syndrome," among others. The clinical features of this syndrome were well described about 50 years ago by Levine and Thompson, who, in turn, referred to the paper by Cuffer and Barbillion, who about 100 years earlier had described "an extra sound appearing a brief interval following the termination of the first heart sound." Pathologic features of this entity were formally described in 1958 by Fernex and Fernex (mucoid degeneration), in 1961 by Oka and Angrist (billowing sail deformity), and in 1965 and 1966 by Read and associates (myxomatous transformation, floppy valve syndrome). A floppy or prolapsed state may involve any of the cardiac valves but is most common in the mitral valve [57].

Prolapse of the mitral valve is now recognized as one of the most common causes of mitral regurgitation. Structurally, the condition is characterized by an increase in the spongiosa layer of the valve leaflets; this layer encroaches upon the fibrosa, causing focal interruptions with lack of support for the valve leaflet.

Two features commonly seen in chronic deforming rheumatic valvular disease, namely commissural fusion and distortion with intrinsic scarring of the valvular tissue, are not usually observed in the myxomatous mitral valve. The changes described lead to prolapse of leaflets into the left atrium [58]. In some cases of mitral valve prolapse, thrombotic lesions may occur in the angle between the ventricular aspect of the posterior leaflet and the atrial wall. Such lesions have been termed *angle lesions*. Among the complications of mitral valve prolapse are ventricular extrasystoles, sudden death, infectious endocarditis, mitral insufficiency, and friction lesions on the ventricular endocardium [59]. Considering that mitral valve prolapse of some degree occurs in nearly 10% of the population, and that sudden death among affected persons is uncommon, it must be concluded that the incidence of sudden death secondary to mitral valve prolapse is very rare [60].

Infectious endocarditis is a recognized complication of mitral valve prolapse. Significant mitral insufficiency can also result from noninfected rupture of mitral chordae. While any element of the mitral valve may be the site of chordal rupture, the most common site is that of one or more chordae inserting into the central scallop of the posterior leaflet. Excessive hooding of the unsupported valvular leaflet occurs with chordal rupture [61–63]; this acts as a baffle, directing the regurgitant blood in a direction opposite to the site of the basis for the valvular insufficiency. Thus, when insufficiency results from rupture of the central scallop of the posterior leaflet, the regurgitant stream is directed medially and strikes that part of the atrial septum lying behind the aortic valve. The resulting systolic murmur may be heard in the aortic area and be confused with aortic stenosis.

Friction lesions tend to occur on the left ventricular endocardium and along chordae of the mitral valve. These fibrous lesions occur in response to friction of unsupported mitral chordae rubbing on the nearby ventricular endocardium. These lesions may be the sites of origin for ventricular premature contractions.

Papillary muscle dysfunction

Myocardial infarction without rupture of papillary muscles may underlie chronic mitral regurgitation. The process has been called *papillary muscle dysfunction*. Scarring or simply ischemia of papillary muscles may be the cause of the mitral insufficiency [64].

The papillary muscles of the left ventricle, the related left ventricular wall, and the anterior papillary muscle of the right ventricle were studied in several conditions associated with left ventricular hypertrophy. Necropsy specimens of hearts without significant coronary disease, from infants or children and adults with a variety of disease states, were studied by Arosemena and associates [64]. The conditions included aortic stenosis, coarctation of the aorta, endocardial fibroelastosis, and left ventricular hypertrophy with congestive heart failure. There was a direct relationship between the severity of fibrosis of the left ventricle and the angiographic demonstration of mitral insufficiency. The common denominator was left ventricular hypertrophy, which appears to be responsible for the scarring of the left ventricular papillary muscles. Mitral insufficiency may result in these cases, with extensive scarring of the left ventricular papillary muscles [65, 66].

In the study of subjects 50 years of age or older, the causes of mitral regurgitation in order of decreasing frequency were myocardial infarction with or without rupture of papillary muscles, rheumatic disease, and infectious endocarditis, as reported by Vlodaver and Edwards [67].

Less common causes were myxomatous mitral valve with noninfected rupture of chordae, calcification of the mitral ring, adhesion of chordae to the left ventricular wall, and cardiomyopathies.

In the normal heart the papillary muscles are oriented vertically. In the failing left ventricle the papillary muscles are turned toward a horizontal position, thereby losing their efficiency. The increased size of the left ventricular cavity also contributes to the size of the mitral orifice [68].

Ergot alkaloid, used in the treatment of migraine headache, and some appetite suppressants have been reported to cause fibrous thickening of the leaflets of the mitral valve and associated mitral insufficiency [69].

Calcification of the mitral ring

Calcification of the mitral ring is very common in the aged. It tends to be more common in women than in men. It rarely causes sudden death except in unusual cases, especially with infection involving the mitral ring. The mitral leaflet may become tethered and entrapped by the calcification. Mitral annular calcification has been described as a marker of severe coronary atherosclerosis in patients less than 65 years of age [70].

Tricuspid regurgitation

The effects of rheumatic fever on the tricuspid valve are similar to those upon the mitral valve but usually lead to tricuspid regurgitation rather than stenosis. In evaluating patients with rheumatic fever, identification of tricuspid regurgitation is generally assumed to represent evidence of rheumatic fever.

In recent years, there has been increased recognition of myxomatous disease of the tricuspid valve, which may occur independently or be associated with myxomatous change of the mitral valve [71]. It is also not uncommon to have tricuspid regurgitation resulting from chordal rupture, which is attributed to past injury [72–75]. Injury to other organs at the time of tricuspid injury had been reported in a case of atrial septal rupture [76], and in a case of traumatic injury to the liver [77]. In a case of tricuspid regurgitation resulting from blunt trauma, a ruptured atrial septum resulted in a right-to-left shunt and persistent systemic hypoxemia [76].

An add uses of tricuspid regurgitation had been associated with systemic lupus erythematosus with or without associated vegetations.

Dilation of the right ventricle, from whatever cause, may be a basis for tricuspid regurgitation. Metastatic carcinoid tumor may result in tricuspid regurgitation and associated pulmonary stenosis. The lesions appear similar to those observed with ergotamine and "fen-phen"-related valve disease [69].

Aortic stenosis

Peterson and associates [78] studied aortic valves that had been removed surgically in 109 cases of aortic stenosis. The following observations were made: The most common type of aortic stenosis requiring surgery was a calcified congenital bicuspid aortic valve [79]; this condition was observed predominantly in male subjects. The second most common type of aortic stenosis was the "senile" type; this is characterized by irregular calcification in the aortic cusps, without any adhesion between the cusps. This type of aortic stenosis was more common in women than in men. The third grouping was that

of rheumatic disease. Either the valve was characterized as an acquired rheumatic bicuspid valve or there was active rheumatic granulation tissue at the commissures.

Regardless of the cause of aortic stenosis, the heart shows significant hypertrophy of the left ventricular wall. In some cases of rheumatic aortic stenosis there are rheumatic changes in other valves, particularly the mitral valve.

Sudden death is not uncommon among patients with aortic stenosis, although other symptoms, such as angina and heart failure, usually predate the development of sudden death.

Complete heart block following replacement of the aortic valve

Studies of hearts with prior aortic valve surgery demonstrated a tendency for conduction disturbance due to the close proximity of the bundle of His and its left branch to the aortic root [80,81]. Fukuda and coworkers [82] reported on 16 cases of complete heart block among 124 patients in whom the aortic valve was replaced by a prosthesis.

The inferior aspect of the noncoronary cusp is closely related to major conduction tissue [83]. During aortic valve replacement, the conduction tissue may be strangulated or injured by sutures, or it may be injured when calcific material of the diseased aortic valve is removed. Complete heart block may also occur as a late manifestation of aortic valve replacement.

Aortic regurgitation

Aortic regurgitation can result from a wide variety of diseases. The process may stem from diseases of the aortic valve, of which there are several; may result from disease of the aortic wall, principally cystic medial necrosis or aortitis; or may be confused with other processes that result in an abnormal escape of blood from the aorta either adjacent to the aortic valve or removed from it [84].

The primary diseases of the aortic valve leading to aortic regurgitation may be congenital or acquired. The congenital diseases are most commonly bicuspid aortic valve although, rarely, quadricuspid aortic valve may also occur and result in aortic insufficiency. Myxomatous prolapse of the aortic valve may lead to significant aortic insufficiency and may be categorized as being congenital in nature [85].

Fenestration of the aortic valve is a very common condition, but aortic regurgitation due to fenestration is rare.

A number of factors may be responsible for prolapse of the semilunar cusps. According to Carter and associates [86] these conditions include intrinsic weakness of the cusp, excessive cuspid tissue, traumatic or infectious diseases of the aortic valvular elements, inadequate support of the aorta as in certain ventricular septal defects, and the loss of commissural support from laceration of the ascending aorta.

Cystic medial necrosis

Cystic medial necrosis is a common condition and it may appear as an isolated entity or be associated with other conditions such as aortic insufficiency, including mitral and/or tricuspid myxomatous disease. Cystic medial necrosis may be a major manifestation of arachnodactyly (Marfan syndrome). Carlson and associates [87] reviewed 250 necropsies with cystic medial necrosis. These were cases with Marfan syndrome, idiopathic dilatation of the aorta, and aortic dissection. The severity of the lesions was graded on a scale of 1 to 4, according to the amount of basophilic ground substance and fragmentation of elastic tissue. According to the authors the incidence of cystic medial necrosis increased with age. Among hypertensive subjects the incidence of cystic medial necrosis was consistently higher than in normotensive subjects.

Spontaneous laceration of the ascending aorta as a complication of cystic medial necrosis may result in loss of commissural support and contribute to aortic insufficiency. Other conditions that may simulate aortic regurgitation are those that cause a diastolic runoff of blood from the aorta into a second area; this would include the ruptured aortic sinus aneurysm or the aortic left ventricular tunnel.

Aortitis

The classical cause of aortic regurgitation due to aortitis is syphilitic aortitis. This condition, fortunately, is less common than in the past. It is characterized by major inflammation of the thoracic aorta, including the ascending aorta, which may contribute to obstruction of the coronary arterial

ostia. The cause of aortic regurgitation is due in part to dilation of the aortic root and separation of the commissures.

Pulmonary stenosis or regurgitation

Pulmonary stenosis may be a complication of rheumatic heart disease. The entity is usually associated with involvement of the other valves by rheumatic disease. The lesion is characterized by nodular thickening at the line of closure of the pulmonary valve. Cardiac involvement with carcinoid syndrome classically includes pulmonary stenosis as well as tricuspid valve disease. Recent studies have shown that the use of the appetite suppressants fenfluramine and phentermine ("fen-phen") may lead to pulmonary stenosis [88].

Significant pulmonary regurgitation is uncommon and generally seen in extreme cases of cystic medial necrosis or in situations with major pulmonary arterial dilatation. The congenital entity of absence of the pulmonary valve may lead to severe pulmonary incompetence early in life.

Infectious endocarditis

Infectious endocarditis may involve any of the valves, but more likely the left-sided valves than the right-sided valves. The disease, which was fatal in the era before the introduction of antibiotics, is now frequently cured by a combination of medical and surgical therapy. Even among cases with fatality, death is not universally sudden. Sudden death from infectious endocarditis may result from cerebral infarct or hemorrhage, coronary embolism, or complete heart block. Endocarditis may occur on native valves, usually with underlying structural abnormalities or on prosthetic cardiac valves [174].

Some unique features of right-sided endocarditis need to be emphasized; namely, fever is commonly absent, murmurs are frequently absent, and the common fatal complication is recurrent septic pulmonary embolism leading to diffuse multifocal infection and infarction of the lung.

In the past it had been taught that rheumatic disease was the classic substrate for infectious mitral valvular endocarditis. The authors are of the opinion that mitral endocarditis occurs more commonly on the myxomatous mitral valve; this may be the result of the declining incidence of rheumatic valvular disease. In the case of aortic endocarditis, congenital disease of the aortic valve, especially congenital bicuspid aortic valve, is a common background.

The bacteremia that leads to infectious endocarditis is often overlooked. Two common conditions underlie the bacteremia that may lead to infectious endocarditis: dental manipulations and urogenital procedures or illnesses. The disease starts on the cusp or leaflet followed by infection of the nearby cusp or leaflet accounting for the "kissing lesion" of early infectious endocarditis. As the disease becomes established a hallmark of infectious endocarditis becomes evident: destruction of valvular tissue, namely cusps and chordae and the presence of valvular vegetations. This process may be followed by secondary foci of infection within the heart, particularly involvement of the mitral valve secondary to primary disease of the aortic valve. In addition to infection within the heart, secondary infections occur anywhere including the central nervous system [89]. In the kidney, infectious endocarditis may be associated with hypersensitivity disease in the form of focal embolic glomerulonephritis ("flea-bitten kidney").

Fungal infections may affect any valve, but more commonly the right-sided valves are involved. The incidence of fungal endocarditis is increasing and may relate to the common use of intravenous drugs and the utilization of long-term indwelling venous catheters. The complications of this process frequently dominate the clinical state of the patient [90].

Indwelling catheter

Becker and associates [91] studied necropsies of patients who had indwelling catheters in the right side of the heart. A bland, noninfectious mural thrombosis was commonly observed. Infection occurred in isolated cases.

Pacemakers and implantable cardioverter-defibrillators have occasionally been associated with heart failure and infection. The clinical presentation can be insidious and difficult to diagnose. Case of *Aspergillus* infection on an implantable cardioverter-defibrillator with right-sided endocarditis are increasingly recognized reported. The infection may be complicated by fungal pneumonia [92].

Marantic valvular vegetation

Marantic valvular vegetations represent one form of nonbacterial endocarditis [93]. The mitral and the aortic valves are the most common sites of involvement. The vegetations are characterized by platelets and fibrin without identification of any microorganisms. Usually, patients with marantic vegetations have an underlying malignant tumor. Systemic arterial occlusion, usually multiple when present, may antedate the identification of the underlying tumor.

Atheromatous (cholesterol) embolism

Eliot and associates [94] reported that crystals of cholesterol (cholesterol embolism) or larger fragments of atheromas (atheroembolism) may be dislodged from ulcerated atheromatous arterial lesions. Such emboli may originate either in the aorta or in any of the major systemic arteries and lodge in small arteries or arterioles. Localized inflammatory response to the foreign body may occur; this reaction may lead to fever and eosinophilia. Atheroembolism may be associated with infarction of visceral organs, especially the kidney and intestines [95].

Atheromatous embolization may result in various clinical presentations ranging from subclinical states to those of obvious arterial occlusion. The occurrence may be spontaneous or may follow arterial catheter manipulation, as in cardiac angiography [96,97]. Myocardial ischemia or infarction, small strokes, cutaneous nodules, renal and splenic infarction, gastrointestinal bleeding, pancreatitis, hypertension, renal failure, and peripheral gangrene are among the clinical manifestations when arteries are occluded by emboli originating in atheromas of the aorta. Syndromes resembling polyarteritis nodosa and bacterial endocarditis may result from widespread cholesterol embolization to small arteries.

Cholesterol embolization should be suspected when the following situations occur simultaneously: pain, fever, livedo reticularis, and intact peripheral pulses [96].

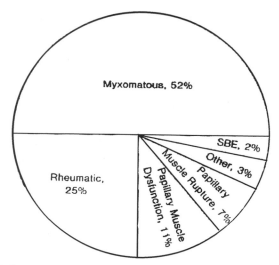

Figure 79 Pathology of surgically excised mitral valves.
Hanson and coworkers analyzed the valves in 100 consecutive cases of mitral valve replacement. Rheumatic mitral valve disease, stenosis, and/or insufficiency accounted for 51% of the cases. Myxomatous changes were present in 32 cases. Nineteen of the latter cases also demonstrated chordal rupture. Four cases demonstrated rupture of papillary muscles secondary to myocardial infarction. In seven cases, papillary muscle dysfunction was the underlying cause requiring mitral valve replacement. In one case, infectious endocarditis was observed. Lupus erythematosus was diagnosed in one case, and miscellaneous causes in two cases.
Reprinted with permission from Hanson and coworkers [52].

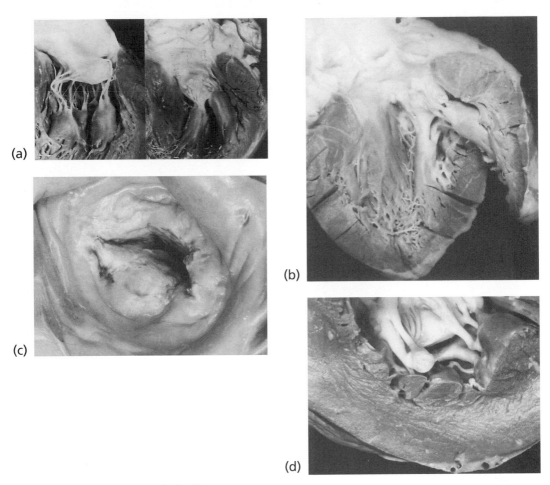

Figure 80 Sudden death due to valvular disease.
Rheumatic mitral disease. Mitral stenosis. (a) Views of the normal (left) and stenotic mitral valve (right). Each viewed from the left ventricle. Female, 68 years (for both). (b) Stenotic mitral valve viewed from inside the left ventricle. There is major cordial fusion. (c) Stenotic mitral valve viewed from above. The orifice is reduced by fibrosis of the leaflets and commissural fusion. (d) Stenotic mitral valve viewed from the left ventricle. The restricted orifice is apparent along with fusion of chordae.

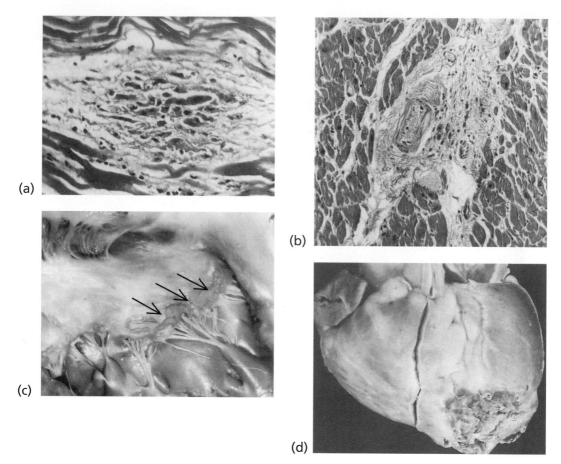

(a)

(b)

(c)

(d)

Figure 81 Background for rheumatic heart disease – acute lesions of rheumatic fever.
(a,b) Photomicrographs demonstrating intramyocardial Aschoff bodies diagnostic of acute rheumatic fever. Females, 20 years and 11 years, respectively. (c) Gross photograph of mitral valve with active rheumatic vegetations along the line of closure (arrow). Female, 20 years. (d) Gross specimen of the heart. Active rheumatic pericarditis. At the site of inflammation the visceral and parietal pericardium were fused. Male, 3 years.

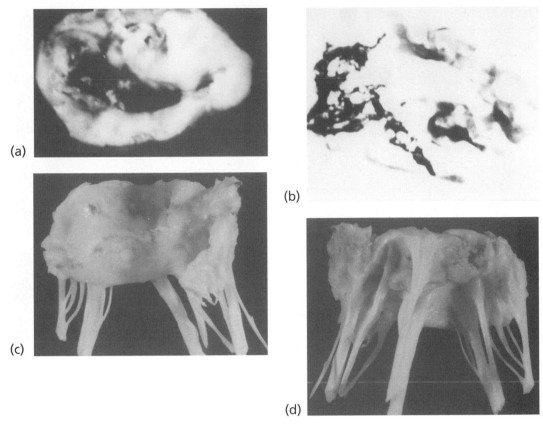

Figure 82 Chronic rheumatic mitral valvulitis with calcification.
Surgically excised mitral valve demonstrating calcification of commissure. (a) Gross photograph of the mitral valve viewed from above. (b) Radiograph of specimen. The dark areas represent major calcification of the anterolateral commissure. Female, 58 years. (c,d) Two views of a rheumatic mitral valve removed surgically demonstrating calcification of leaflets with calcification and fusion of chordae.

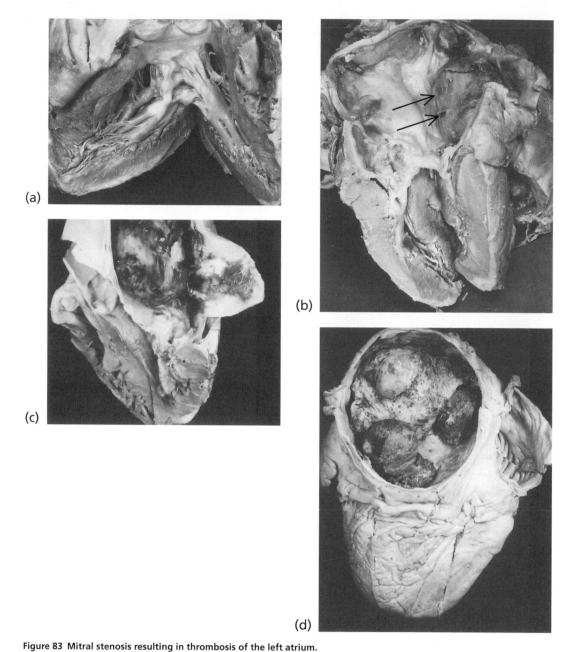

Figure 83 Mitral stenosis resulting in thrombosis of the left atrium.
(a) Rheumatic mitral stenosis viewed from left ventricle, there is scaling of the mitral valve with commissural and chordal fusion . (b) Mitral stenosis as viewed from the left side of the heart. Major narrowing of the mitral orifice is seen with a mural thrombus in the left atrium (arrows). (c) Left side of heart with mitral stenosis. Multiple thrombi in the left atrium including one of major size attached to the wall. (d) Interior of left atrium viewed from posterior, in a case of mitral stenosis. There is dilation of the left atrium with massive thrombosis sudden death. Male, 60 years.

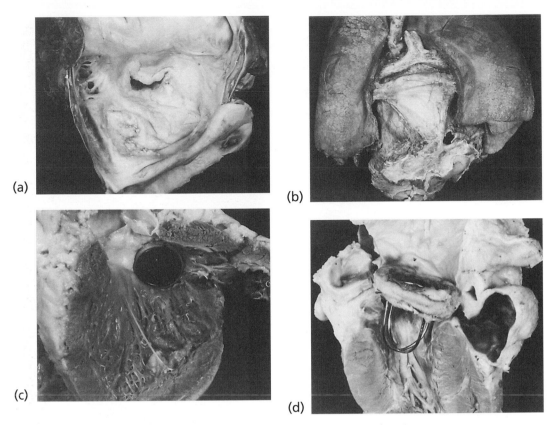

Figure 84 (a,b) Enlarged left atrium of mitral stenosis increases angle of tracheal bifurcation.
(a) Interior of left atrium from above showing mitral stenosis. (b) Thoracic organs viewed from behind. Enlarged left atrium causes an increase in the angle of tracheal bifurcation. In this setting the enlarged left atrium may compress the left recurrent laryngeal nerve causing unilateral vocal cord paralysis. Female, 31 years.
(c,d) Mitral valve replacement injury to the left ventricle.
(c) Interior of left ventricle following replacement of stenotic mitral valve by a prosthetic valve. A perioperation tear in the left ventricle caused death of the patient. Female, 75 years. (d) Left side of heart, with a mitral valve prosthesis having been replaced about 5 years previously, associated with a false aneurysm (arrows) of the left ventricle. The latter lesion is considered to be a complication of the original operation. Female, 61 years.
Reprinted with permission from Joassin and Edwards [159].

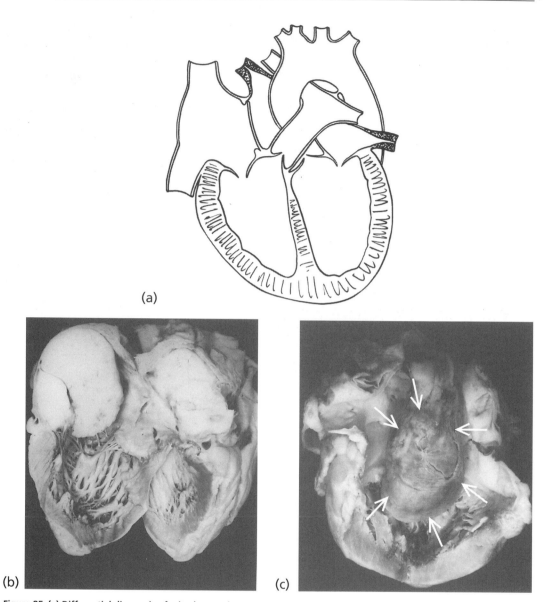

(a)

(b)

(c)

Figure 85 (a) Differential diagnosis of mitral stenosis.
Diagrammatic representation of stenosis of pulmonary veins. Although incomplete, the following list of differential diagnoses of mitral stenosis or insufficiency pertains: (1) left ventricular failure (primary), (2) left ventricle obstruction by thrombus, (3) parachute mitral valve, (4) supravalvular mitral ring, (5) hypereosinophilic syndrome, (6) pulmonary veno-occlusive disease, (7) stenosis of pulmonary veins, (8) left atrial myxoma, (9) left atrial sarcoma, and (10) cor triatriatum.
Reprinted with permission from Edwards [109].
(b,c) Pulmonary venous obstruction by malignant tumor.
(b) Filling of the left atrium by left atrial sarcoma. Female, 26 years. (c) A segment of a pulmonary vein; a tumor causing luminal obstruction is attached. The tumor extends through the left atrium and into the left ventricle. The tumor (arrows) was an undifferentiated tumor of pulmonary origin. Female, 74 years.

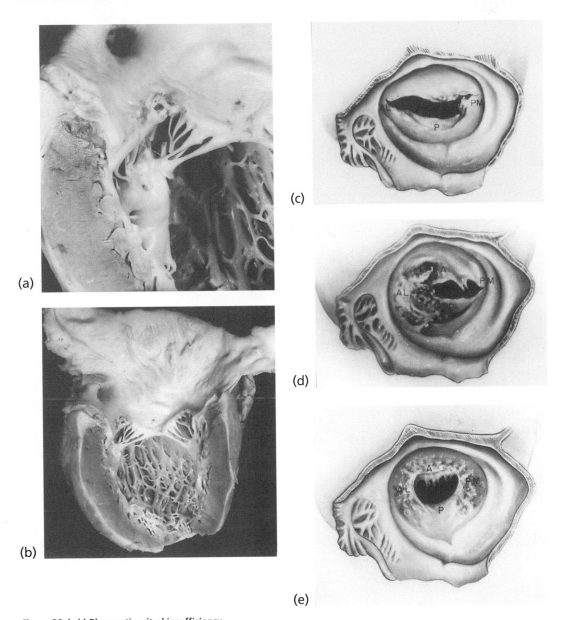

Figure 86 (a,b) Rheumatic mitral insufficiency.
(a) Early stage of rheumatic mitral insufficiency with thickening of some chordae and minor fusion of the commissure.
(b) Established rheumatic mitral insufficiency. The left atrium is enlarged. The posterior leaflet shows thickening at the junction of the closing edge. The endocardium of the left ventricle is thickened.
(c,d,e) Diagrammatic presentation of three types of rheumatic mitral insufficiency.
(c) Simple type. (d) One commissure is normal. The other is scarred; the "dew drop" type of mitral insufficiency. (e) Both commissures are fused and the leaflets are shortened, leading to the "wedding ring" type of deformity.

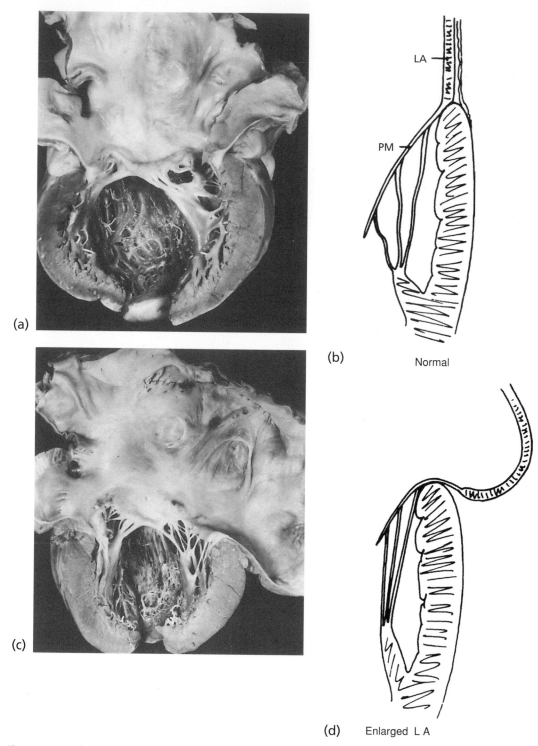

(a)

(b)

Normal

(c)

(d)   Enlarged L A

Figure 87 "Mitral insufficiency begets mitral insufficiency."
(a) Mild rheumatic mitral insufficiency with normal left atrial size. The mitral valve is in a normal position.
(b) Diagrammatic illustration of the relationship between the left atrium and mitral valve in the normal state. (c) Severe rheumatic mitral insufficiency with marked left atrial enlargement. The dilation of the left atrium pulls the posterior leaflet of the mitral valve over the base of the left ventricle thereby, accentuating the degree of mitral insufficiency.
(d) Diagrammatic illustration of the displacement of the posterior leaflet of the mitral valve in patients with left atrial enlargement.
Reprinted with permission from Edwards and Burchell [161] and Edwards [162].

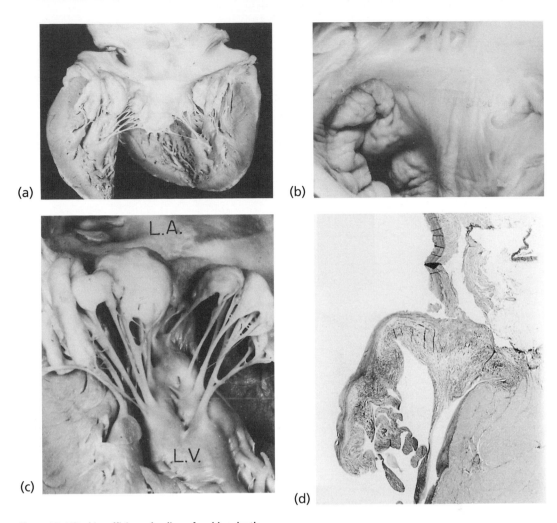

(a)

(b)

(c) L.A. L.V.

(d)

Figure 88 Mitral insufficiency leading of sudden death.
Myxomatous mitral valve. (a) Classic example of myxomatous mitral valve primarily involving the posterior leaflet.
Dilation of the left atrium and left ventricle is consistent with mitral insufficiency. This degree of prolapse, though rare,
may be associated with sudden cardiac death. Female, 25 years. (b) The mitral valve is unopened and viewed from above.
Both the anterior leaflet (right side of illustration) and the posterior leaflet (left side of illustration) show prominent
hooding or "floppiness." Female, 25 years. (c) Gross photograph of a myxomatous mitral valve with prominent
interchordal hooding of units of the valve. (d) Photomicrograph showing thickening of the left ventricular endocardium.
This has resulted from injury to the endocardium by contact with the mitral valve and chordae during the cardiac cycle.
Female, 25 years.
Reprinted with permission from Edwards [163].

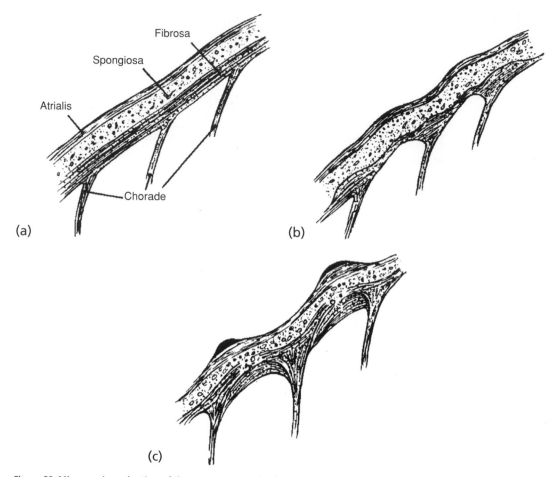

Figure 89 Microscopic evaluation of the myxomatous mitral valve.
Diagrammatic illustration of the histologic appearance of the normal mitral valve and the mitral valve with myxomatous change as a guide to the photomicrographs illustrated in Figure 90. (a) The normal mitral valve. The layers of the valve are indicated. (b) In the early changes of the myxomatous mitral valve there is an increase in both the fibrosa and atrialis layers. (c) The changes of myxomatous mitral valve are prominent by irregular thickening of the atrialis layer and further thickening of the fibrosa layer.

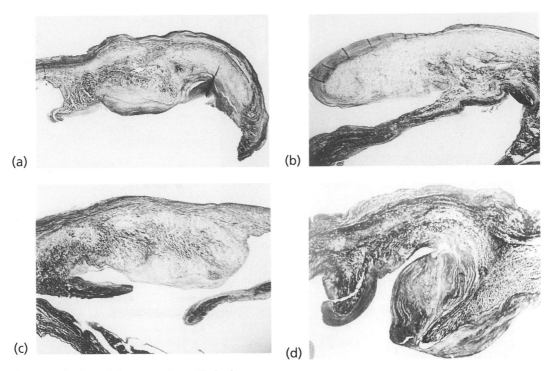

Figure 90 Histology of the myxomatous mitral valve.
The various changes include an increase in the spongiosa layer with varying degrees of thickening of the layers facing the atrium and ventricle. The illustrations are representative of changes frequently seen in myxomatous mitral valve.

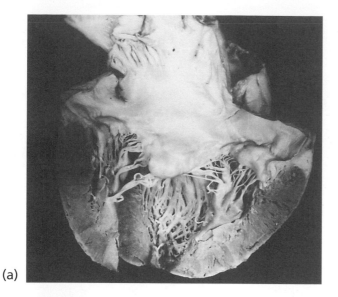

(a)

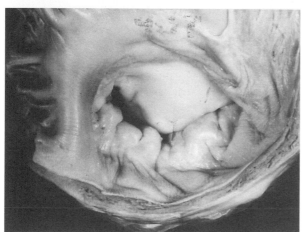

(b)

Figure 91 Mitral insufficiency due to myxomatous mitral valve.
Mitral regurgitation may occur in the myxomatous mitral valve because of simple deformity, or complications such as cordial rupture. The case considered here shows an incompetent mitral valve, without associated complications. (a) Left side of heart. The anterior leaflet is mildly deformed. The posterior leaflet has numerous areas of hooding with prolapse into the left atrium. (b) Close-up view of unopened mitral valve from above. The posterior leaflet shows numerous units with interchordal hooding; the left part of the anterior leaflet is also deformed. The left side of the valve seems to be the major site of mitral regurgitation. Male, 79 years.

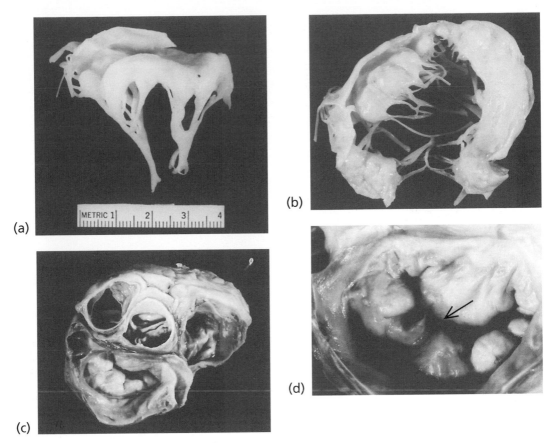

(a)

(b)

(c)

(d)

Figure 92 (a,b) Spontaneous rupture of chordae.
While the myxomatous mitral valve is susceptible to infectious endocarditis with rupture of mitral chordae and onset or accentuation of mitral regurgitation, spontaneous rupture of chordae may complicate the myxomatous mitral valve without infection. The degree of mitral insufficiency may vary depending on the extent of rupture. (a) Surgically excised mitral valve with chordal rupture. (b) A surgically excised valve with mitral prolapse and spontaneous rupture of chordae attached to the anterior leaflet. Male, 66 years.
(c,d) Case of myxomatous mitral valve with ruptured chordae near the central part of the posterior leaflet.
(c) The base of the heart viewed from above. Prominent hooding of the mitral valve is seen. (d) The mitral valve (close-up view). The stump of the ruptured chord is seen near the center of the posterior leaflet (arrow).
Reprinted with permission from Edwards [57].

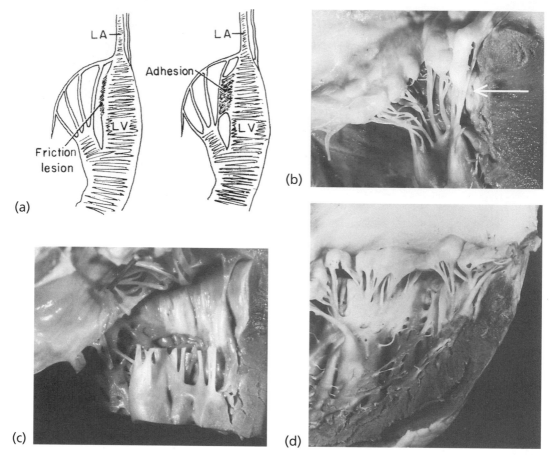

Figure 93 Traumatic lesions of the endocardium resulting from the myxomatous mitral valve.
(a) *Left*: Diagram of the mitral valve and chordae. A friction lesion has started on the surface of the chord nearest to the ventricular endocardium. *Right*: A stage beyond that shown in the left. The reaction over the chord has created an adhesion between the chord and the mural endocardium. (b) In a specimen with (arrow) myxomatous mitral valve, fibrous adhesions are interposed between the chordae and the mural endocardium. (c) In a myxomatous mitral valve the chordae to the posterior leaflet have been cut to allow a clear view of the chordal adhesions to the ventricular wall.
(d) Myxomatous mitral valve. There is widespread thickening of the left ventricular mural endocardium and incorporating chordae of the mitral valve. This irritation of the endocardium may predispose to ventricular arrhythmias and may be one of the mechanisms causing sudden death in patients with mitral valve prolapse. Female, 27 years.
Reprinted with permission from Salazar et al. [59].

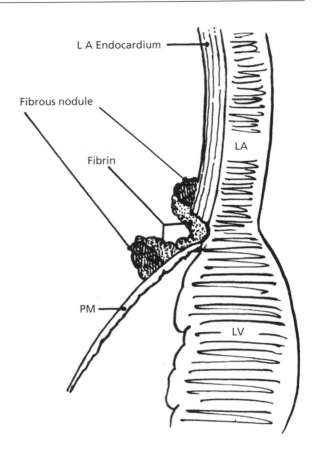

L A Endocardium

Fibrous nodule

Fibrin

LA

PM

LV

(a)

Figure 94 Myxomatous mitral valve "angle lesion."
(a) Diagrammatic view of the posterior leaflet of the mitral valve and surrounding structures. There are fibrous deposits in the angle between the left atrial endocardium and the surface of the posterior mitral leaflet. The composite of the illustration shown may be called the *angle lesion*. These lesions may be a source for emboli. (b) Illustration of the posterior wall of the left atrium and the posterior leaflet of the mitral valve. The leaflets show features of myxomatous mitral valve. The narrow black line above the mitral leaflets is the angle lesion (arrows). Female, 74 years.
Reprinted with permission from Edwards [57].

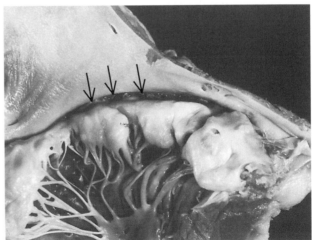

(b)

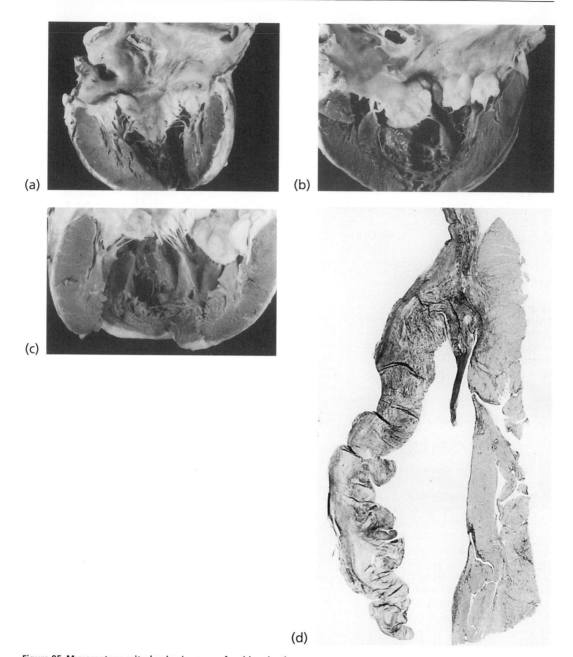

Figure 95 Myxomatous mitral valve in cases of sudden death.
Three cases. (a) Left atrium, left ventricle, and entire mitral valve. The valve shows myxomatous change. Male, 35 years.
(b) Mitral valve showing mostly the posterior leaflet. The atrial septum shows a small defect. Female, 27 years. (c) The
classical myxomatous mitral valve, gross photograph. (d) Photomicrograph of the posterior mitral leaflet. Both (c) and
(d) are from a 36-year-old female in whom sudden death occurred.
Reprinted with permission from Pocock et al. [164].

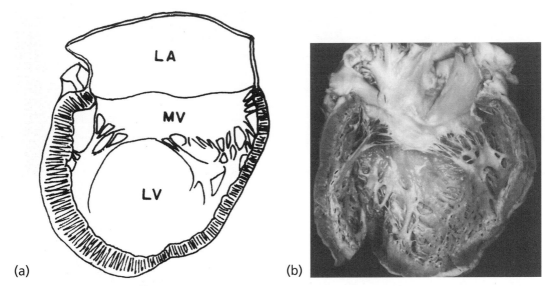

(a)   (b)

Figure 96 Papillary muscle dysfunction leading to mitral insufficiency.
(a) Drawing showing remodeling of the myocardium following acute myocardial infarction. The posteromedial papillary muscle has lost support from the underlying myocardium and the geometry of the two papillary muscles has changed.
(b) Illustration of left side of heart showing atrophy and fibrosis of posteromedial papillary muscle from healed infarction. Subendocardial myocardial infarction may be the cause of mitral insufficiency, one cause of "papillary muscle dysfunction."

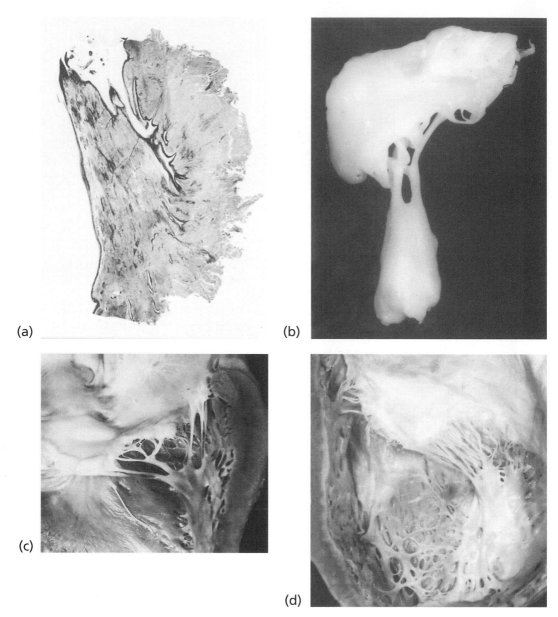

(a)   (b)

(c)   (d)

Figure 97 Papillary muscle disorders causing mitral insufficiency.
(a) Low-power photomicrograph of left ventricle and a papillary muscle showing multifocal scars from healed myocardial
infarction. Female, 3 months. (b) Segment of the mitral valve and attached rupture of one unit of a papillary muscle.
(c) A papillary muscle and related mitral valve showing scarring of the papillary muscle. Male, 35 years. (d) Left ventricle
and a scarred papillary muscle of healed myocardial infarction. Male, 56 years.
Reprinted with permission from Lee et al. [165].

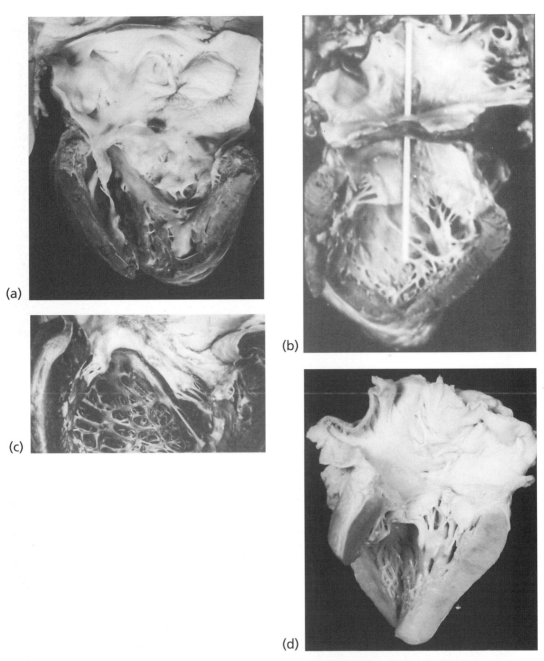

Figure 98 Unusual conditions to be entertained in a differential diagnosis of mitral stenosis or insufficiency.
(a) Left side of heart in corrected transposition with incompetence of the left atrioventricular (AV) valve. Left atrium dilated secondary to insufficiency of the left AV valve. This is an example of corrected transposition with situs solitus; thus the valve is an inverted tricuspid valve lying between the left atrium and the right ventricle, which propels blood into the aorta. Male, 82 years. (b) Cor triatriatum. Left atrium is divided into upper and lower chambers. The probe extends from the upper to the lower chamber through a congenital perforation of the membrane separating the two. Male, 21 days. (c) Mitral insufficiency resulting from a congenital cleft in the anterior leaflet of the mitral valve. (d) Hurler's syndrome. The left atrium is pale; the mitral valve is serrated.

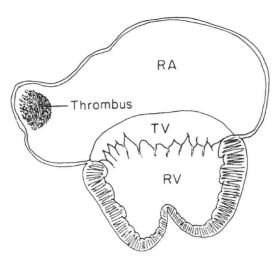

Figure 99 Tricuspid regurgitation.
Diagrammatic representation of the right side of the heart in tricuspid regurgitation with a thrombus in the right atrial appendage.

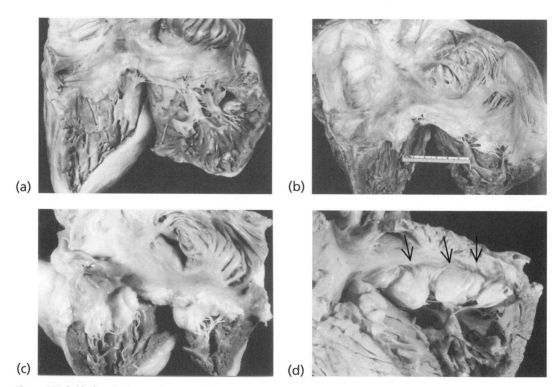

(a)

(b)

(c)

(d)

Figure 100 (a,b) Chronic rheumatic tricuspid regurgitation.
Features of chronic rheumatic tricuspid regurgitation. Illustration on right portrays more advanced lesions than the illustration on the left. There is shorting of the chordae. The right atrium and ventricle are enlarged.
(c,d) Myxomatous tricuspid valve leading to tricuspid regurgitation.
(c) Gross photograph of tricuspid valve with myxomatous change. There is intrachordal hooding, giving prominent cleftlike appearance to the leaflets. Male, 86 years. (d) Myxomatous tricuspid valve with "angle lesion" (arrows). Male, 50 years.

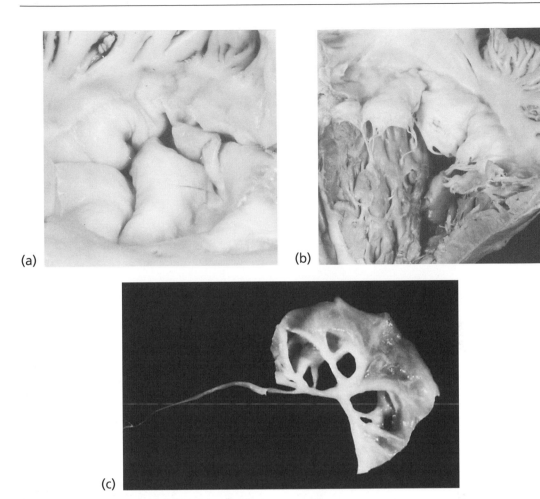

(a)

(b)

(c)

Figure 101 (a,b) Tricuspid regurgitation in a case of pulmonary emphysema.
(a) Unopened tricuspid valve and portion of right atrial appendage. The tricuspid valve shows deformities characteristic of myxomatous change. (b) Details of myxomatous change of opened tricuspid valve. There is prominent right ventricular hypertrophy.
(c) Ruptured chordae of tricuspid valve (probably traumatic) with chronic tricuspid regurgitation.
Ruptured chordae of tricuspid valve in a 65-year-old man with chronic tricuspid regurgitation.

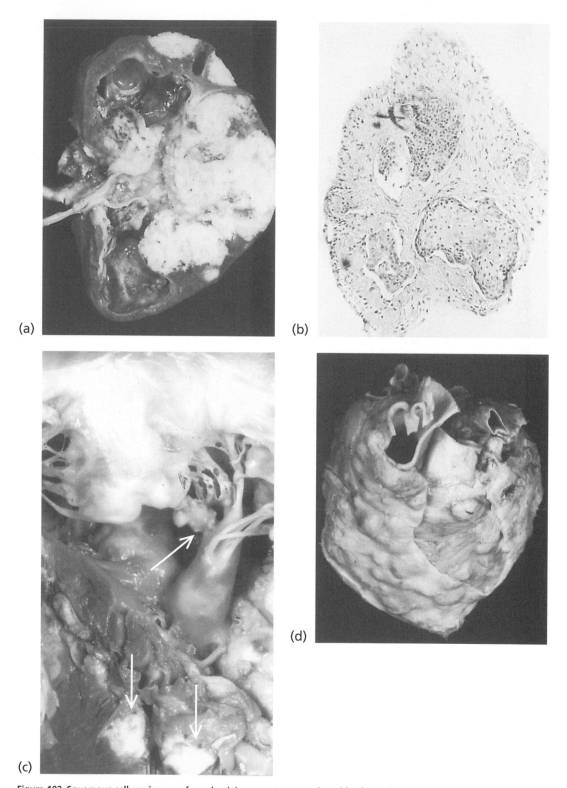

Figure 102 Squamous cell carcinoma of renal pelvis; metastases to tricuspid valve and pericardium.
(a) Kidney with tumor. (b) Photomicrograph of primary tumor showing squamous cell carcinoma. (c) Metastatic carcinoma to papillary muscles of chordae of tricuspid valve (arrows). (d) Metastatic carcinoma to pericardium.

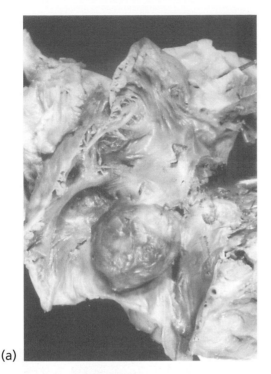

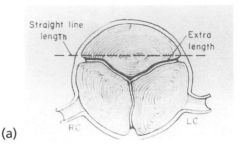

(a)

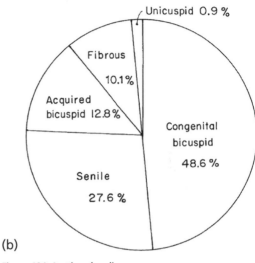

(b)

Figure 104 Aortic valve disease.
(a) Diagrammatic view of the aortic valve from above. Each cusp shows "extra length." The extra length has a dual purpose: it allows the orifice to be closed during diastole and wide open during systole. (b) Distribution of major types of aortic stenosis in a survey of aortic valves that were removed surgically.
Reprinted with permission from Peterson et al. [78].

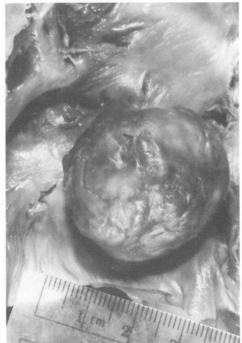

(b)

Figure 103 Tricuspid orifice obstruction by right atrial myxoma.
(a) Right atrium and ventricle, as well as tricuspid valve. A triangular mass obstructs the orifice of the tricuspid valve. (b) Close-up view of the right atrial myxoma lodged in the tricuspid orifice. This obstruction to ventricular filling may result in sudden death. Female, 64 years.

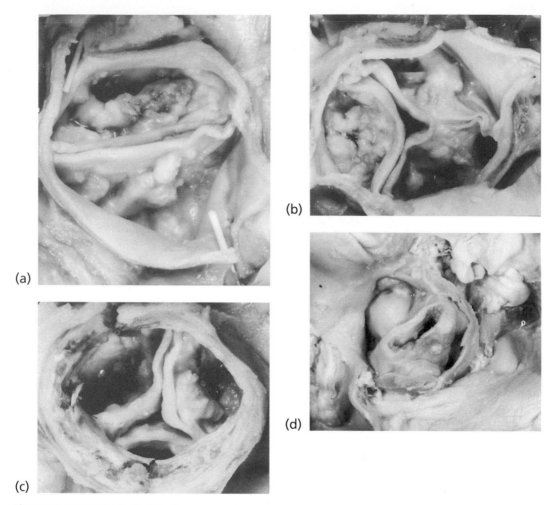

Figure 105 Aortic stenosis: The big three.
(a) A classical example of calcified bicuspid aortic valve. A probe is in each coronary ostium. (b) Rheumatic bicuspid aortic valve. A fused commissure showing the two aortic cusps in the left side of the illustration. (c) "Senile calcified aortic stenosis." The cusps are calcified, but the commissures are not fused. (d) Unicuspid congenital aortic stenosis – an uncommon addition to "the big three" causes of aortic stenosis. All types of aortic stenosis can present as sudden death.

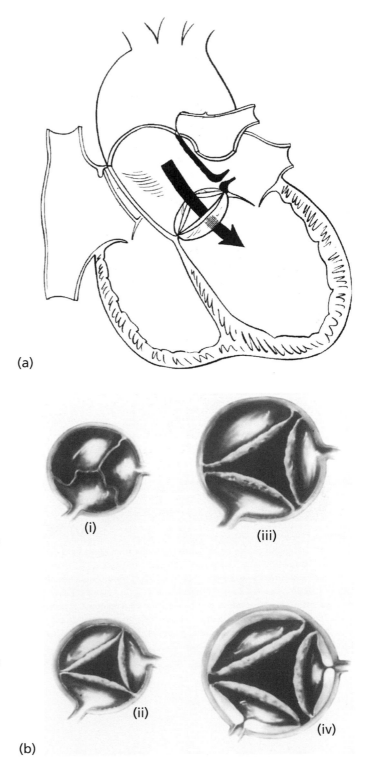

Figure 106 Aortic regurgitation. Aortic regurgitation may develop from disease in the valve or in the wall of the ascending aorta. A large variety of conditions may simulate aortic regurgitation because of runoff of blood from the aorta. (a) A diagrammatic view of aortic regurgitation. Some forms of aortic regurgitation such as syphilitic aortitis may have coexistent coronary ostial stenosis as illustrated. (b) Diagrammatic view of the aortic valve rendered incompetent by several background diseases. (i), Normal; (ii), rheumatic endocarditis as a cause of aortic regurgitation; (iii), aortic insufficiency in cystic medial necrosis; (iv), aortic insufficiency in syphilitic aortitis.

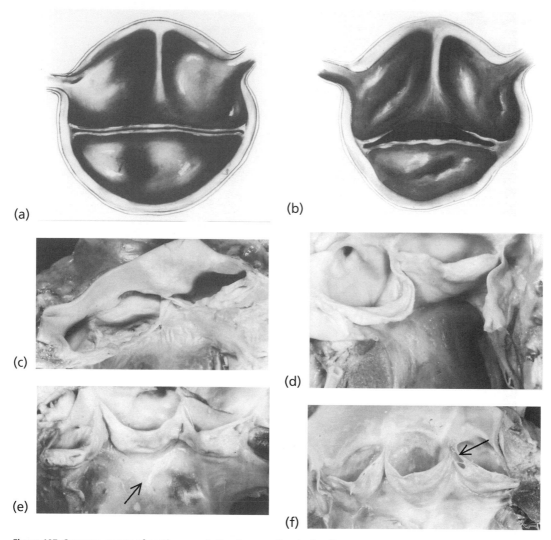

Figure 107 Common causes of aortic regurgitation from aortic valvular disease.
(a) A diagrammatic view of a congenital bicuspid aortic valve. (b) Diagrammatic view of congenital bicuspid aortic valve with aortic insufficiency. The conjoined (larger) cusp shows retraction associated with aortic regurgitation. (c) Congenital bicuspid aortic valve. The conjoined cusps receive a raphe and are deformed. The cusp is poorly supported, leading to incompetence. (d) Myxomatous aortic valve. One cusp demonstrates prolapse beneath an ostium of a coronary artery. Male, 75 years. (e) Rheumatic aortic insufficiency with scarring and contraction of the cusps. There is a subaortic jet lesion seen on the left ventricular endocardium (arrow). (f) Fenestration of aortic cusp (arrow). This is an unusual cause of significant aortic insufficiency.

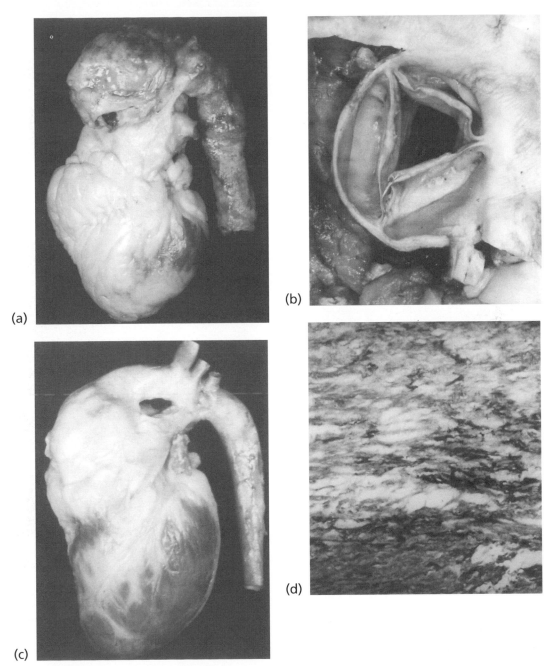

Figure 108 Common causes of aortic regurgitation from disease of the aortic wall.
(a) External view of the heart and thoracic aorta. Syphilitic aortitis with aneurysmal dilatation of the ascending aorta.
(b) The aortic valve cusps are attenuated because of dilation of the aorta; this is a case of syphilitic aortitis. (c) Cystic medial necrosis of the aorta in a patient with Marfan syndrome. Major dilation of ascending aorta. Male, 21 years.
(d) Photomicrograph of aorta showing severe cystic medial necrosis. Male, 13 years.
Reprinted with permission from Edwards [84].

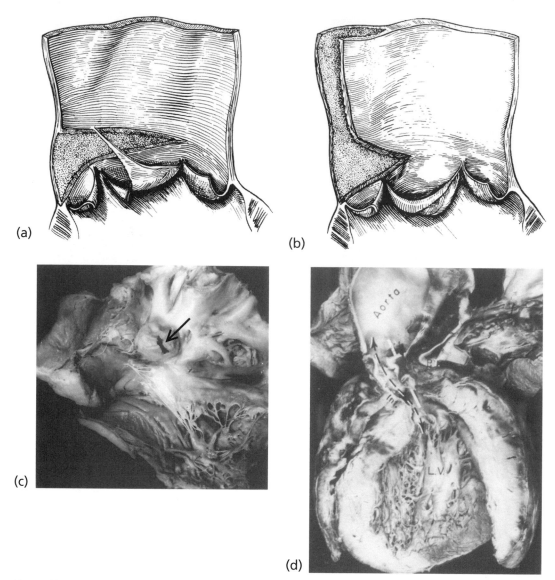

Figure 109 Common causes of aortic regurgitation from disease of the aortic wall.
(a) Spontaneous laceration of ascending aorta with rupture and distortion of the aortic cusps. (b) Classic example of type I aortic dissection with involvement of ascending aorta and secondary aortic insufficiency. (c) Right atrial view of ruptured aneurysm of the posterior aortic sinus (arrow) resulting in an aortic right atrial fistula and wide pulse pressure simulating aortic insufficiency. (d) Congenital aortic left ventricular tunnel. A channel (arrow with dashed lines) runs beside the dilated ascending aorta from the aortic wall, bypassing the aortic valve and entering into the left ventricle. Male, 5 years. Reprinted with permission from Edwards [84] and Levy et al. [166].

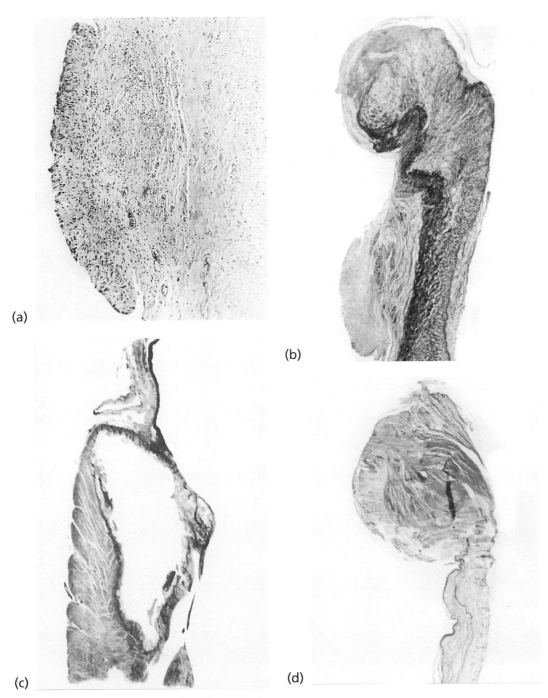

Figure 110 Pulmonary valvular stenosis of rheumatic origin.
(a) The pulmonary valvular Aschoff body consistent with acute rheumatic fever. (b) The free end of a pulmonary cusp with fibrosis and thickening of the valve secondary to a cellular infiltrate. There is loose connective tissue deposited on the valve. The latter is interpreted as fibrosis of rheumatic origin. Female, 4 years. (c) Low-power photomicrograph. The pulmonary trunk and pulmonary valve. The valve was calcified and considered to be a form of pulmonary stenosis of rheumatic origin. A calcific focus extends into the wall of the right ventricle. (d) A chronic deformity of the pulmonary valve. The free edge of the valve is thickened with dense collagen capped by looser connective tissue as a result of rheumatic inflammation. Female, 60 years.

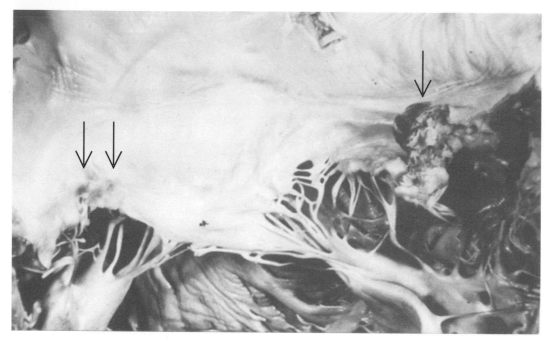

Figure 111 Infectious endocarditis affecting the mitral valve.
Opened mitral valve showing two foci of infectious endocarditis. The lesion on the right (single arrow) is the primary site of infection and the lesion on the left (double arrow) is considered a secondary infection from contact with the first lesion during the cardiac cycle. The secondary lesion is the "kissing lesion."

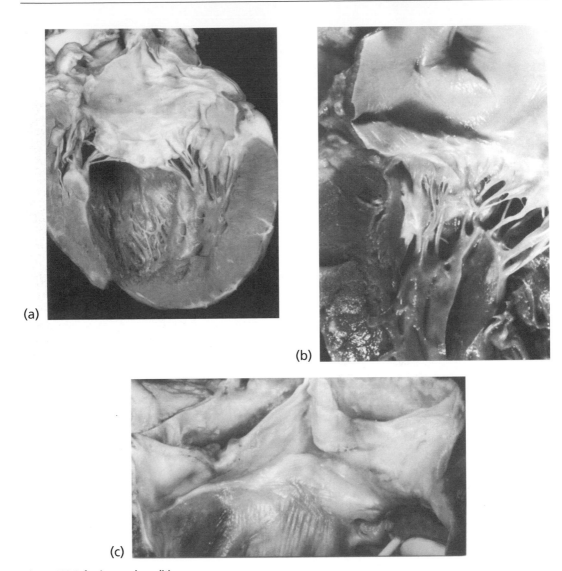

(a)

(b)

(c)

Figure 112 Infectious endocarditis.
Background for infectious endocarditis. Myxomatous valve. (a,b) Two examples of myxomatous mitral valve; the latter condition is more commonly recognized now than in the past. The illustration to the left shows posterior leaflet of the mitral valve to be broken by many pseudocommissures. The illustration to the right shows a myxomatous valve with subvalvular adhesions to chordae. *Left*, female, 70 years; *right*, male, 73 years. Reprinted with permission from Salazar and Edwards [59]. (c) A congenital bicuspid aortic valve. The aortic valve shows laxity of the cusps and a subaortic jet lesion on the surface of the subjacent ventricular septum. Male, 67 years.

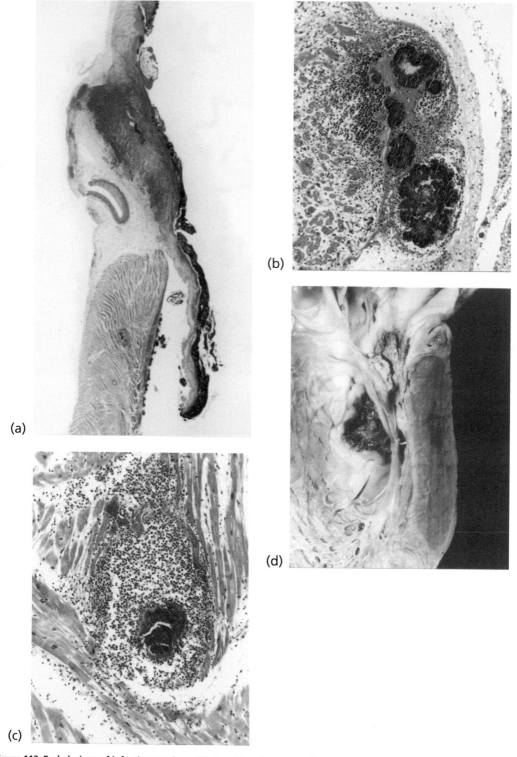

Figure 113 Early lesions of infectious endocarditis involving the myocardium.
(a) Endocarditis of the right atrium, tricuspid valve, and right ventricular myocardium. Vegetations are present on the tricuspid leaflet. Leukocytic infiltrate. Male, 49 years. (b) Right ventricular myocardium and endocardium. Extensive acute inflammatory activity. (c) Myocardial abscess containing a colony of bacteria. (d) Dissecting abscess from left ventricle to left atrium. Male, 85 years.

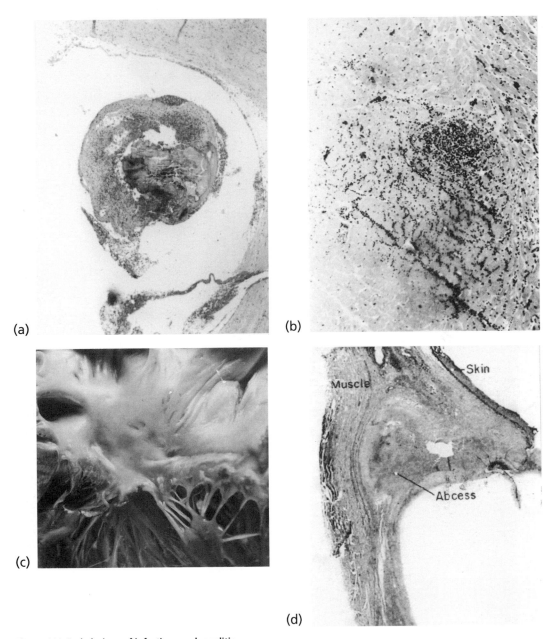

Figure 114 Early lesions of infectious endocarditis.
(a) A coronary embolus composed of vegetations from a valve with endocarditis. Male, 56 years. (b) Myocardium with hemorrhage and inflammation as a complication of early infectious endocarditis. Male, 56 years. (c) Early rupture of the mitral chordae secondary to endocarditis. (d) Metastatic abscess in the leg of a patient with infectious endocarditis. Reprinted with permission from Dry et al. [167].

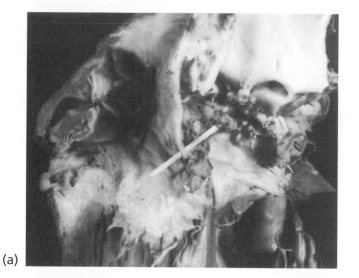

(a)

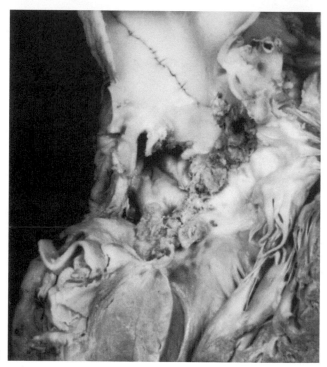

(b)

Figure 115 Complete heart block complicating infectious endocarditis.
In a study by Wang and coworkers of 142 cases of infectious endocarditis, complete heart block was found in 6 cases and first-degree or second-degree atrioventricular block in 14 cases. Among the 20 cases with atrioventricular (AV) disturbance, the aortic valve was involved in 18.
(a) Severe destructive aortic endocarditis with a fistula to the right atrium (probe). The destruction is in the vicinity of the AV node causing complete heart block. (b) Another example of aortic endocarditis in continuity with the atrioventricular node. Male, 63 years.
Reprinted with permission from Wang et al. [83].

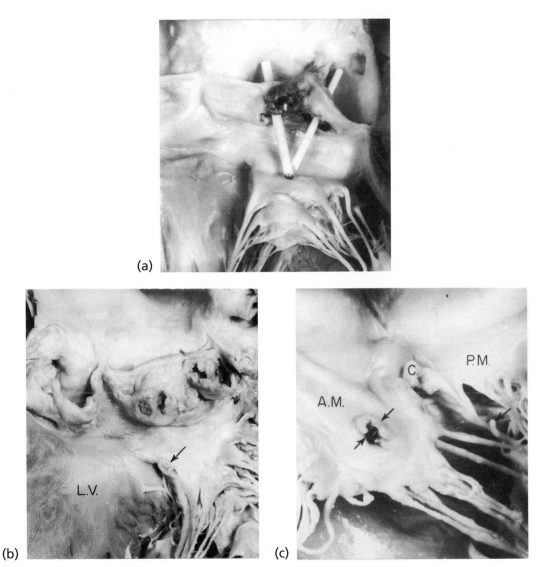

Figure 116 Primary aortic valvular endocarditis may become complicated by infection of the subjacent mitral valve.
(a) The aortic valve is the site of infectious endocarditis with two perforations in the valve. Each perforation contains a
probe aiming toward the subjacent mitral valve. Male, 65 years. (b) Aortic valve perforations from infectious endocarditis.
Arrow points to secondary endocarditis of the mitral valve. L.V., left ventricle. (c) The anterior leaflet (A.M.) of the mitral
valve shows a perforation (between arrows). P.M., posterior leaflet of the mitral valve; C., commissure between anterior
and posterior leaflets.
Reprinted with permission from Edwards [168].

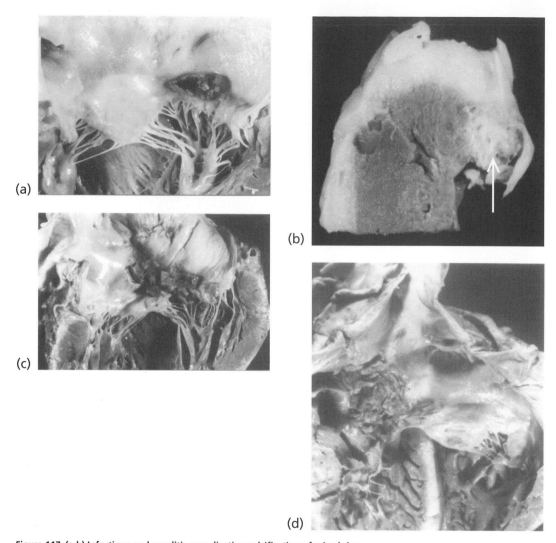

(a)

(b)

(c)

(d)

Figure 117 (a,b) Infectious endocarditis complicating calcification of mitral ring.
(a) Endocardial view of left atrium and mitral valve. The lesion represents a vegetation of infectious endocarditis including involvement of subjacent mitral ring. (b) Base of left ventricle and mitral ring containing inflammatory lesion (arrow).
(c,d) Simultaneous infection of multiple valves.
(c) Mitral valve; site of active infectious endocarditis. (d) Right side of heart in the same case. The tricuspid valve is the site of infectious endocarditis.

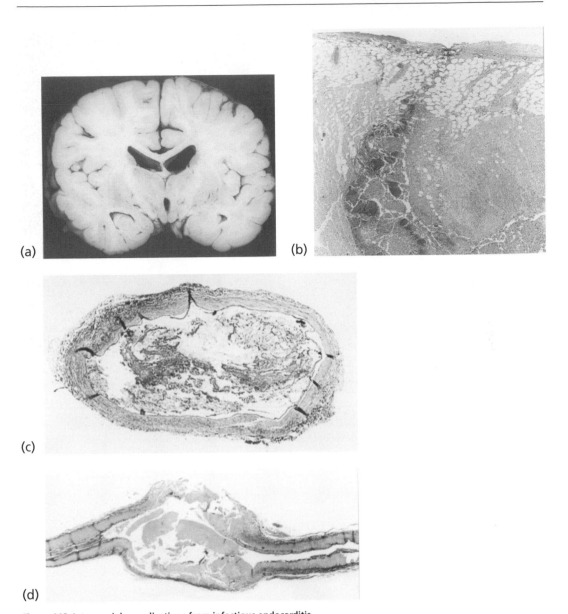

Figure 118 Intracranial complications from infectious endocarditis.
(a) Cerebrum. Infarction of the right cerebral cortex from emboli. Male, 68 years. (b) Metastatic soft tissue abscess in case from (a). (c) Right middle cerebral artery. Lesions secondary to infectious endocarditis. The wall of the artery is thickened with heavy leukocytic infiltration. The lumen contains an infected thrombus. Male, 44 years. (d) A cerebral artery showing a segment of acute arteritis in a patient with endocarditis. Male, 42 years.

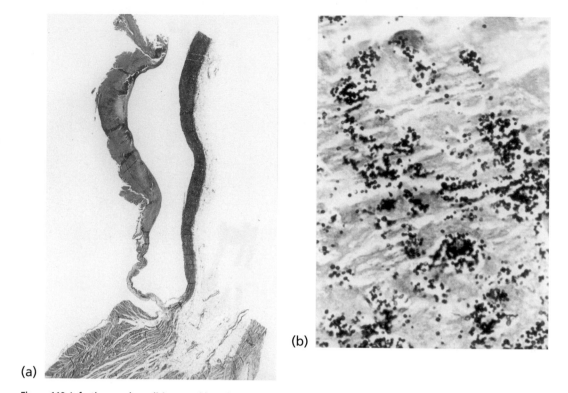

(a)

(b)

Figure 119 Infectious endocarditis caused by a fungus.
Pulmonary valve in endocarditis from fungus. (a) Low-power photomicrograph of pulmonary valve and wall of pulmonary trunk. The valve is swollen and contains organisms of the infectious agent. (b) Photomicrograph. Fungal organisms in the pulmonary valve.

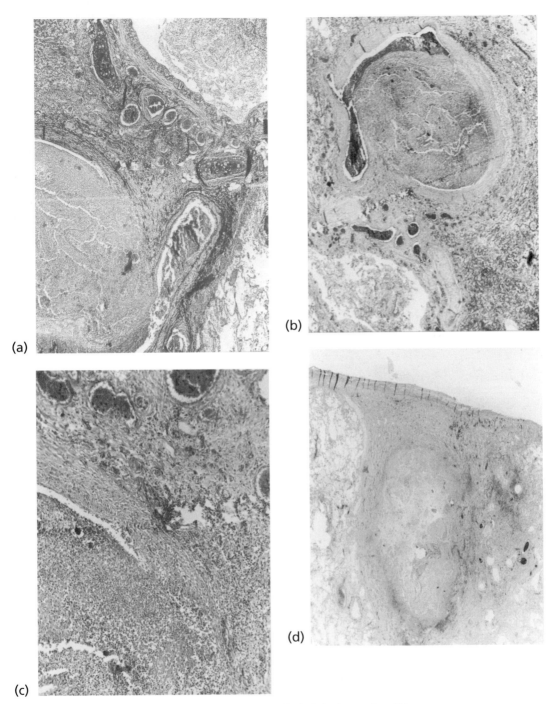

Figure 120 Pulmonary embolism in tricuspid or pulmonary valvular infectious endocarditis.
In contrast to left-sided endocarditis in which the brain, the heart, and the kidney are frequent sites of embolic complications, infections of the right-sided valves lead to pulmonary complications in the form of emboli containing the infectious organism. (a,b) Lung showing embolism of infectious material. (c,d) Angitis and pneumonia with abscess formation in the lung.

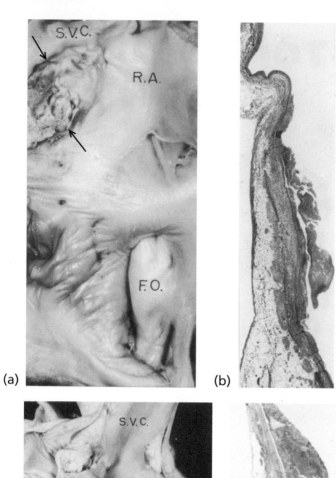

(a)

(b)

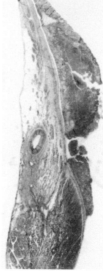

(c)

(d)

Figure 121 Infectious endocarditis in relation to intracardiac catheter.
(a) Mural thrombus at the junction of the superior vena cava and right atrium secondary to an indwelling cardiac catheter (between arrrows).
(b) Photomicrograph of mural thrombus shown at left. No infectious agents were identified. (c) Interior of junction of superior vena cava (SVC) and right atrium (RA) shows a pedunculated thrombus, which developed in a patient who had a long-standing venous catheter. (d) Photomicrograph of specimen shown at left. A thrombus is attached.
In both (c) and (d), numerous blastospores of *Candida* were present. Reprinted with permission from Becker et al. [169].

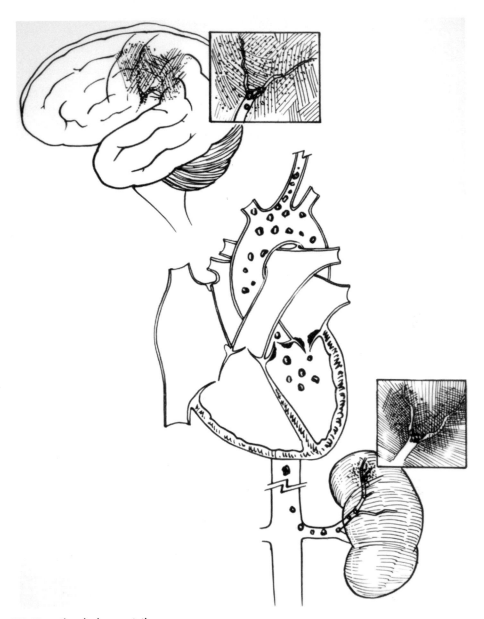

Figure 122 Marantic valvular vegetations.
Diagrammatic portrayal of systemic embolism from marantic vegetations from the mitral and aortic valves. Marantic valvular vegetations represent one form of nonbacterial endocarditis. The mitral valve and aortic valve are the most common sites associated with marantic vegetations. Multiple systemic arterial occlusions may antedate the identification of an underlying malignant tumor.
Reprinted with permission from Becker et al. [169] and Waller et al. [170].

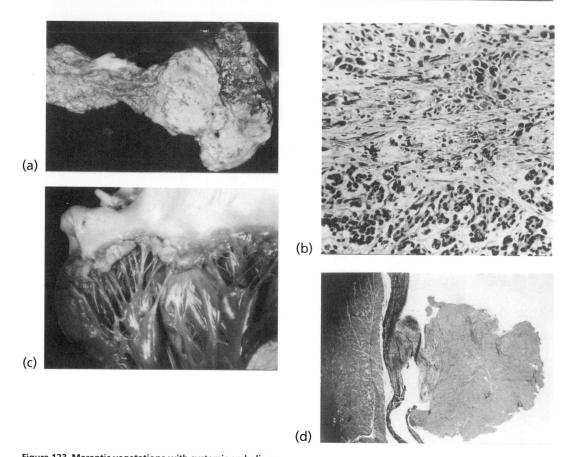

Figure 123 Marantic vegetations with systemic embolism.
(a) The pancreas showing adenocarcinoma in the tail. (b) Histologic view of the pancreatic carcinoma. (c) Mitral valve with marantic vegetations; the latter are bulky and subject to fragmentation and embolism. (d) Photomicrograph of marantic vegetation. Sterile emboli were found in the coronary arteries and other systemic arteries.
Reprinted with permission from Becker et al. [169].

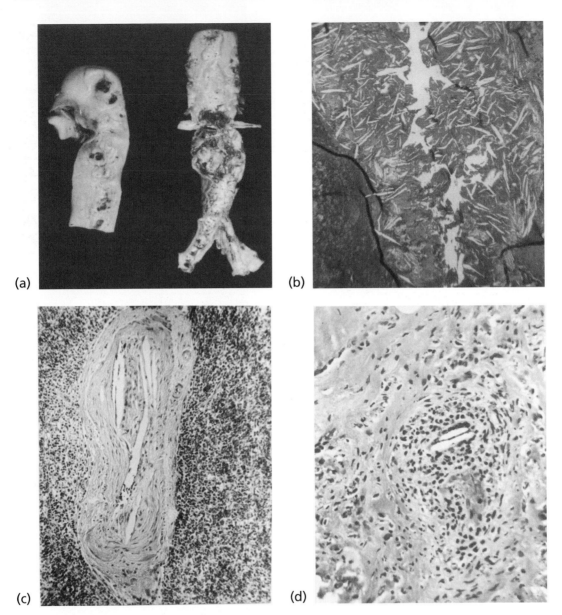

Figure 124 (a,b) Cholesterol (atheromatous) embolism.
(a) The thoracic and abdominal aortae. Severe atherosclerosis.
(b) Low-power photomicrograph of portion of aortic atherosclerosis; multiple cholesterol crystals.
Reprinted with permission from Eliot et al. [94].
(c,d) Illustration of small arteries containing cholesterol emboli.
(c) Small artery cut in longitudinal section. (d) Inflammatory leukocytic reaction to the presence of sites of cholesterol embolic crystals.

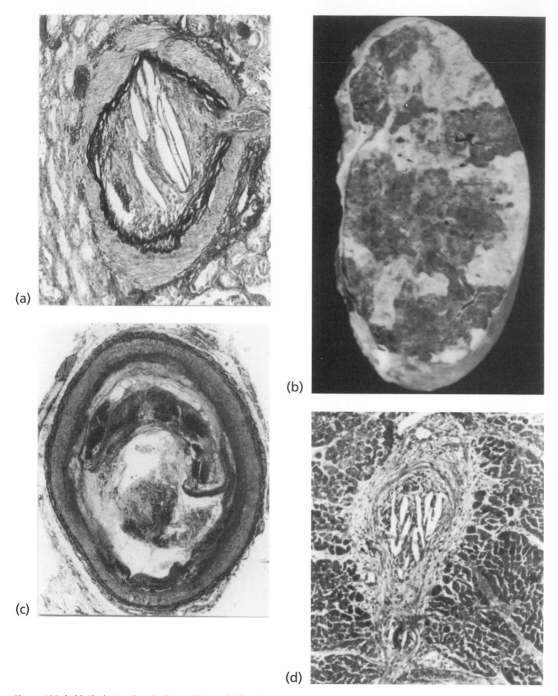

Figure 125 (a,b) Cholesterol embolism with renal infarction.
(a) Photomicrograph of the kidney. The kidney is one of many sites of cholesterol embolism. (b) Gross specimen: infarction of kidney secondary to a shower of cholesterol emboli from a highly diseased aorta.
(c,d) Cholesterol embolism starting in a coronary artery.
(c) A coronary artery showing atherosclerosis with cholesterol crystals in the lumen of the artery. (d) Section of myocardium. Interstitial artery contains numerous cholesterol crystals. Coronary arteries may be a primary site of cholesterol embolization, as shown in this pair of illustrations. Involvement of a coronary artery may also be secondary to embolization from aortic atherosclerosis.

CHAPTER 7

Metabolic and infiltrative disorders

There are many substances, carbohydrates, proteins, metals, and whole cells, which may infiltrate various organs including the cardiovascular system. The authors have chosen a limited number of conditions namely sarcoidosis, amyloidosis, and glycogen storage disease to be presented in this book. All these conditions can be associated with sudden death.

Sarcoidosis

Sarcoidosis is an inflammatory disease (cause not isolated) that affects lungs, lymph nodes, myocardium, and other organs. In the myocardium the lesion tends to be granulomatous with a varying number of multinucleated giant cells. Cardiac sarcoidosis has been reported masquerading as right ventricular dysplasia or isolated atrioventricular block [98–101]. Syncope and sudden death may occur in patients with sarcoidosis [102]. Okura and associates [103] presented a clinical and histopathologic report on an investigation in which they compared clinical data to assess the association between histologic appearance and survival. The purpose was to determine whether histologic features could differentiate between giant cell myocarditis and sarcoidosis. Transplant-free survival is better for patients with sarcoidosis than for those with giant cell myocarditis. Presentation with heart failure predicted giant cell myocarditis, and presentation with heart block predicted sarcoidosis.

Amyloidosis

Amyloidosis is a heterogeneous group of disorders resulting in deposition of proteins in the extracellular space of various tissues and organs. There are several types of amyloid disease now classified by the nature of the precursor proteins that form the amyloid deposits. AL amyloidosis is the result of deposition of immunoglobulin light chain in various

tissues. Cardiac involvement is very common, and death is usually the result of congestive heart failure or arrhythmia. AL amyloidosis is the result of a plasma cell dyscrasia related to multiple myeloma. Familial amyloidosis is the result of a non-plasma cell derived fibular protein, transthyretin (TTR). Many mutations of transthyretin have been recognized, but the most common mutation is known as transthyretin amyloidosis (ATTR). The protein is produced by the liver but is deposited in many extra hepatic sites, including heart, peripheral nerves, gastrointestinal tract, and skin. Secondary type of amyloid infiltration, known as SAA amyloid, is the result of deposition of the acute phase reactant "serum amyloid A" in response to chronic inflammation resulting from disorders such as tuberculosis, chronic osteomyelitis, rheumatoid arthritis, and inflammatory bowel disease.

Senile amyloid tends to occur in the elderly and results from transthyretin deposition. It tends to involve the atria primarily [104], although it may infiltrate all portions of the heart and the lung. Usually the senile amyloid does not result in functional impairment. Valvular amyloid is a rare manifestation of senile amyloid in which the infiltrate primarily affects the cardiac valves; valve function is usually not severely affected [105].

AL amyloid: primary systemic amyloid

Primary systemic amyloid represents a plasma cell disorder with abnormal production of kappa or lambda light chains. The light chains may infiltrate many organs [106]. Cardiac and renal failures are common [107]. In certain situations patients may undergo stem cell transplantation with or without solid organ transplantation of the heart or kidney [107]. Once they become symptomatic with heart failure, patients may deteriorate quickly and die of progressive congestive heart failure or sudden death. Grossly the heart has thick, firm walls and a waxy coloration. Diastolic dysfunction may result in large atria and occurs before the onset of systolic dysfunction. Histologically the myocytes appear encased by the amyloid protein, which appears bright with congo red staining. Vascular staining is also commonly observed.

Glycogen storage disease

Glycogen storage diseases are a heterogeneous group of conditions that may present at any time from infancy to adulthood. There is not cardiac involvement in all forms of glycogen storage disease. Lysosomal acid maltase deficiency is also known as glycogen storage disease type II. If present during infancy, it is known as Pompe disease and is associated with cardiomyopathy and early death. Juvenile and adult forms are recognized and usually not associated with cardiomyopathy. The condition is characterized by deposits of glycogen in lysosomes and cytoplasm. Glycogen deposits are seen in the interstitial tissues of the liver and the heart and in the skeletal muscles [108].

Hemochromatosis

Hemochromatosis is a hereditary disorder characterized by abnormal intestinal iron absorption. Once absorbed, the iron is initially deposited in the liver. Only after hepatic iron storage is saturated does significant cardiac iron accumulate. Once overloaded with iron, the heart displays significant systolic dysfunction and dilatation. Without the aid of special iron stains, hemochromatosis of the heart may be mistaken for a dilated cardiomyopathy. Cardiac hemochromatosis however does not occur without coexistent hepatic cirrhosis. Sudden death may occur with advanced hemochromatosis.

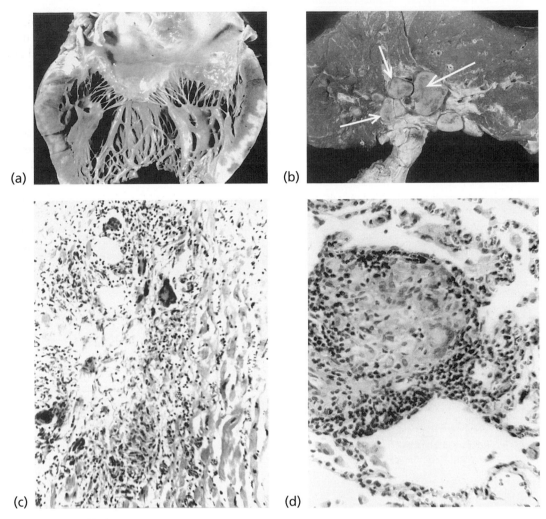

(a)

(b)

(c)

(d)

Figure 126 Sarcoidosis.
Classical example; male, 25 years. (a) Left ventricular wall shows intramyocardial focal nodules of sarcoidosis on the cut surface of the left ventricle. (b) Hilum of lung showing prominently enlarged lymph nodes, the sites of sarcoid granulomas (arrows). (c,d) Low-power and high-power photomicrographs of myocardium showing granulomas containing Langerhans' giant cells.

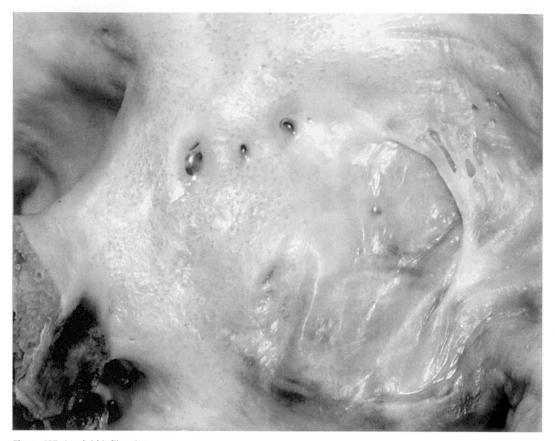

Figure 127 Amyloid infiltration.
Gross photograph of the endocardial surface of the left atrium showing the stippled effect of amyloid infiltration.

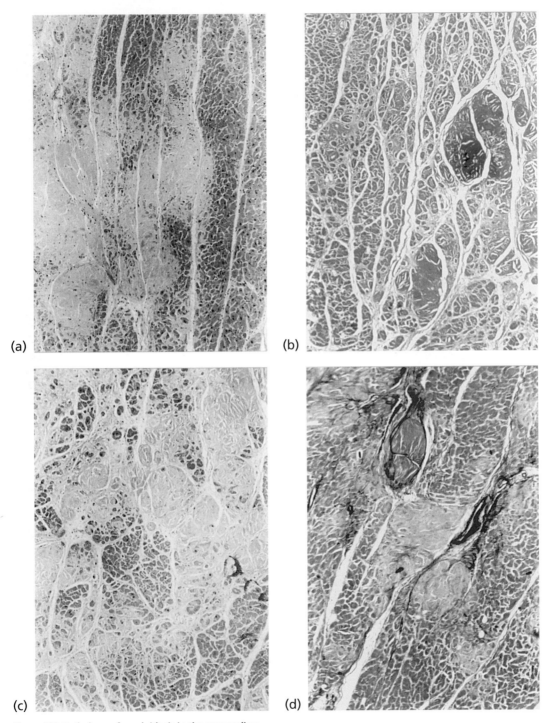

Figure 128 Pathology of amyloidosis in the myocardium.
(a,b) Foci of amyloid in the myocardium. The amyloid protein tends to surround myocytes. Amyloid may exist in nodules as seen in the right. (c,d) Two examples of amyloid infiltration in the myocardium. The process is diffuse. While the H&E stains are suggestive of amyloid, confirmation usually requires specific staining such as congo red stain. Male, 77 years.

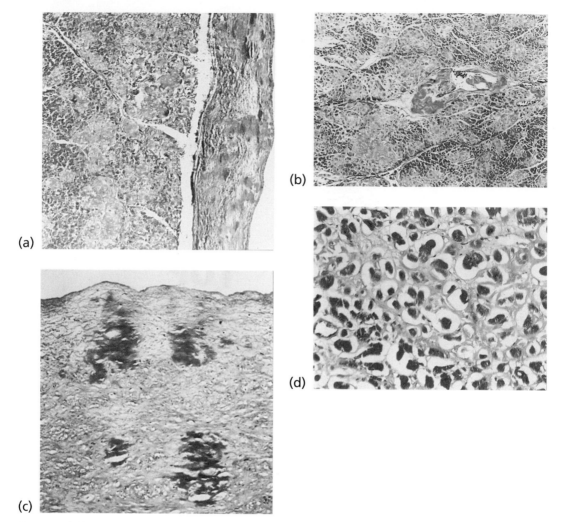

(a)

(b)

(c)

(d)

Figure 129 (a,b) Systemic amyloidosis with severe cardiac enlargement.
Male, 88 years. (a,b) Multiple areas of amyloid infiltration into the myocardium. The sites of involvement may be large and associated with myocardial atrophy.
Reprinted with permission from Layman et al. [171].
(c,d) Major amyloid infiltration with myocardial atrophy.
(c) The amyloid infiltration tends to be focally distributed. (d) The infiltration of amyloid is followed by atrophy of the involved cells ("amyloid rings"). The amyloid surrounds myocytes and "insulates" them, thereby producing the characteristic low voltage on ECG.

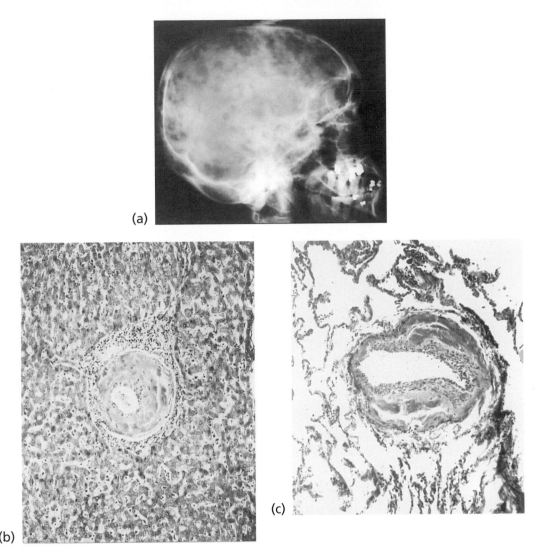

Figure 130 Systemic features of amyloidosis.
Male, 88 years. (a) Multiple myeloma; radiograph of a patient with numerous skeletal erosions. (b) Photomicrograph showing vascular amyloid infiltration in the liver. (c) Lung. An artery is narrowed by amyloid infiltrating its wall. Reprinted with permission from Layman et al. [171].

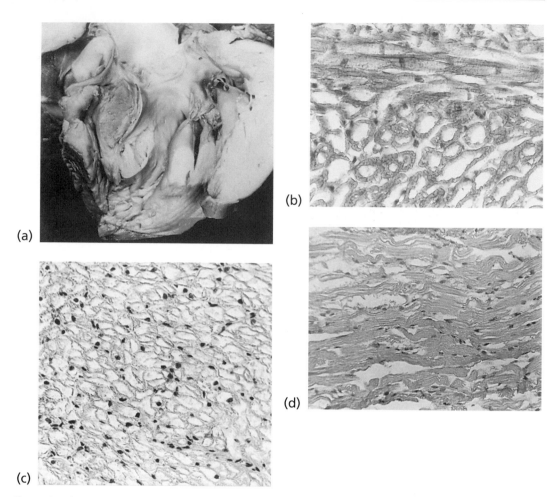

Figure 131 Glycogen storage disease.
Muscles of the heart and skeletal system may be infiltrated in glycogen storage disease, causing atrophy of muscles with corresponding weakness of myocardium and of the skeletal system. (a) The myocardium in glycogen storage disease. The myocardium is pale, with increased wall thickness. Male, 7.5 months. (b) Photomicrographs of myocardium. There are prominent vacuoles in the myocardial fibers caused by glycogen storage disease. Male, 7.5 months. (c) Photomicrograph of liver showing major vacuolization of hepatocytes due to glycogen deposition. Male, 3 months. (d) Skeletal muscle showing the vacuolization of skeletal muscle fibers. Male, 3 months.
Reprinted with permission from Ruttenberg et al. [108].

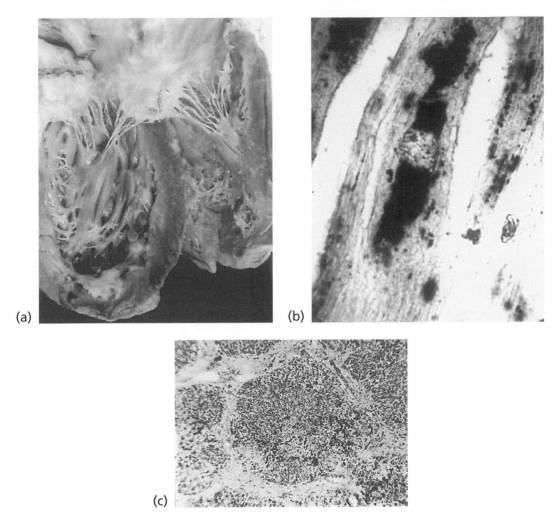

(a)

(b)

(c)

Figure 132 Hemochromatosis.
Abnormal intestinal uptake of iron is the cause of hemochromatosis. Deposits in the myocardium result in myocardial failure. Male, 45 years. (a) Left side of heart. The myocardium is discolored by the accumulation of hemosiderin in the interstitial myocytes. Grossly the left ventricle may have the appearance of a dilated cardiomyopathy. (b) Photomicrograph of the myocardium stained for iron. The positive stain for iron is characteristic of the brown of the myocardium. (c) Photomicrograph from liver showing pigment cirrhosis. Male, 33 years.

CHAPTER 8

Tumors and blood dyscrasias

Cardiac tumors, both primary to the heart and metastatic, may cause sudden death [109,110]. Death may be the result of direct tumor infiltration, arrhythmias, space occupancy, or obstruction of blood flow.

Primary tumors of the cardiovascular system

Myxomas

Myxomas occur in either atrium, more commonly in the left atrium than in the right atrium. Myxomas have two major potentials for disability or death. One is fragmentation, leading to disseminated emboli, which may cause infarction of various organs or death. Another major cause of death is either obstruction or major stenosis of blood flow due to tumor involvement in the related atrioventricular valve. Experience has shown that when the tumor is removed, the attachment to the atrial septum should also be removed so as to avoid a local recurrence of the tumor. Some myxomas may have a genetic basis, such as those that occur as part of the Carney complex, which is characterized by multiple cardiac myxomas, lentiginosis, and endocrine dysfunction.

Mesothelioma of the atrioventricular node

Mesothelioma of the atrioventricular (AV) node is usually a small benign tumor, which may escape pathologic recognition unless careful examination of the region of the AV node is undertaken. Although the tumor behaves as a "benign" neoplasm, it may have "malignant" implications causing complete heart block and sudden death. It tends to occur more frequently in females [111].

Pericardial teratoma

Usually seen in children, the pericardial teratoma is a retrosternal tumor. As the name implies, the tumor has several identifiable tissues often including tissue from all three germ lines.

Rhabdomyoma of the ventricles

Rhabdomyoma is represented by one large mass causing major obstruction and death in infancy. Rhabdomyomatosis and diffuse rhabdomyomatosis are related conditions. The tumor is rare and shows foci of benign giant cells infiltrating the myocardium. Shrivastava and associates [112] present the case of a seemingly well 13-year-old boy who died suddenly. The myocardium was infiltrated by cells like those of classical congenital rhabdomyoma of the heart. In contrast to the latter condition, in which distinct nodules are present, their patient had an infiltrated myocardium without a distinct tumor formation. This may be designated as *diffuse rhabdomyomatosis*.

Angiosarcoma of the heart

This highly malignant tumor may arise in the heart or pericardium, often showing a predilection for right-sided structure including the right atrium and right ventricle. Often, but not universally, there is an intracavitary portion of the tumor that may lead to obstruction of blood flow or interference with valve function. The tumor is highly aggressive with widespread metastases that are not very responsive to therapy. Hemorrhage into the pericardium from this highly vascular tumor may cause cardiac tamponade and death.

Noncardiac tumors affecting the cardiovascular system

Noncardiac tumors may affect the cardiovascular system by a variety of mechanisms. The tumor may act as a space-occupying lesion, obstructing venous return to the heart, or may infiltrate the myocardium itself. Metastatic disease to the pericardium is especially common and may result in diastolic dysfunction or frank cardiac tamponade. Cardiac arrhythmias, including atrial fibrillation, occur commonly with metastatic disease to the pericardium. The conduction system may occasionally be primarily affected by a metastatic tumor. We have observed an adult patient with complete heart block in whom sudden death occurred. The autopsy showed a malignant tumor involving the bundle of His; the primary site was not identified. Metastatic tumors that frequently affect the heart include breast, lung, melanoma, and primary hematologic malignancies.

Carcinoid heart disease is reviewed in Chapter 11.

Blood dyscrasias

Several conditions classified as blood dyscrasias are reviewed in the illustrative part of this book. These include aplastic anemia with hemorrhagic foci; polycythemia with hemorrhages involving the pericardium; and thrombotic thrombocytopenic purpura, resulting in both thrombosis and hemorrhage.

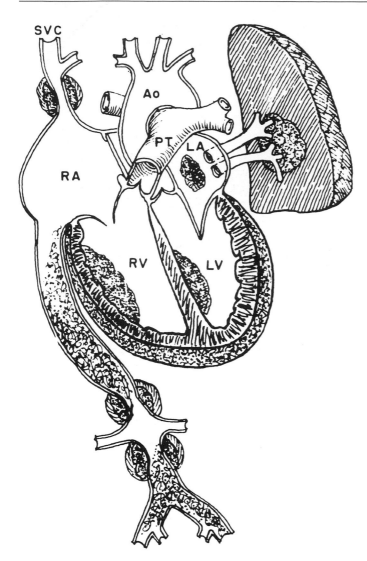

Figure 133 Tumors affecting the heart and great vessels.
Tumors affecting the cardiovascular system may be either primary or secondary. Secondary tumors affect the heart in mechanical ways yielding obstruction to flow or encasement of the heart. This illustration demonstrates the variety of ways tumors can affect the heart and great vessels, including caval obstruction, myocardial or pericardial infiltration, inflow or outflow obstruction, and pulmonary venous obstruction among other disorders. Reprinted with permission from Edwards [109].

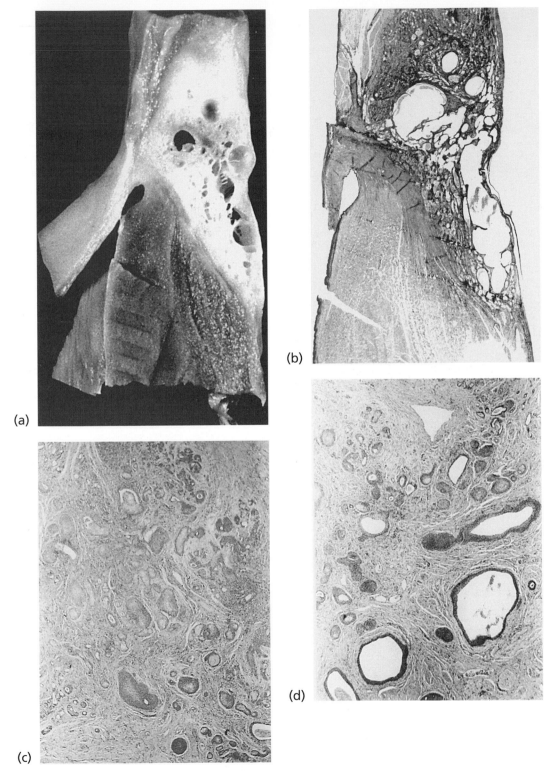

(a)

(b)

(c)

(d)

Figure 134 Primary tumors of the heart. Mesothelioma of the atrioventricular node.
Complete heart block is commonly seen in patients with mesothelioma of the atrioventricular (AV) node because of
its effect on conduction tissue. Female, 51 years. (a) Gross specimen of the right atrium and right ventricle in the region
of the AV node. There is a cystic-appearing mesothelioma of the AV node. (b) The tumor has progressed downward into
the right ventricle. (c) Photomicrograph of portions of the tumor. The tumor has a tendency for glandular formation.
(d) Photomicrograph of portions of the tumor. Some of the glands are cystic.
Reprinted with permission from Ibarra-Perez et al. [47].

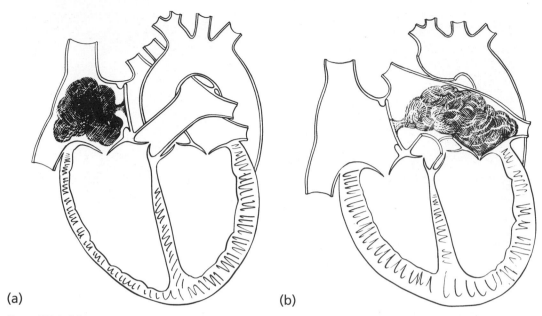

(a)   (b)

Figure 135 Atrial myxomas.
Atrial myxomas may develop in either right- or left-sided chambers. Sometimes, especially when familial, they may be multiple. (a) Myxoma of right atrium with its characteristic point of attachment at the atrial septum. (b) Myxoma of left atrium causing mitral inflow obstruction.

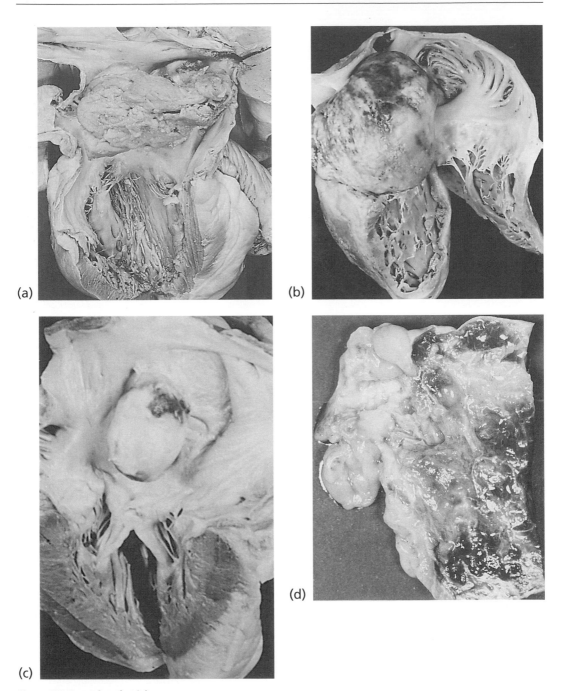

Figure 136 Examples of atrial myxomas.
(a) Tumor involving left atrium and extending through the mitral valve, causing major obstruction. Female, 13 years.
(b) Right atrial myxoma causing major crowding of the right atrium. The atrium is enlarged. (c) A case of left atrial myxoma that has calcified. Female, 87 years. (d) Surgical specimen of a left atrial myxoma. Tumor is large and friable. In addition to being a space-occupying lesions that may limit blood flow, these types of myxomas may be especially prone to embolization. Male, 72 years.
Reprinted with permission from Tiffany et al. [172] and Carter et al. [173].

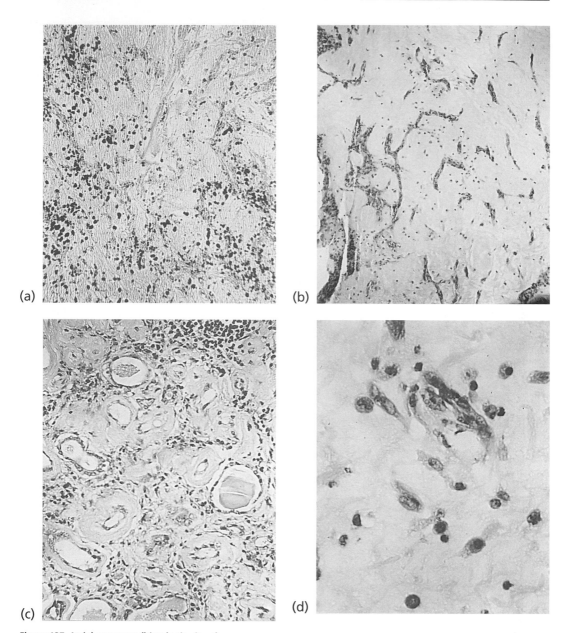

Figure 137 Atrial myxomas (histologic views).
Histologic appearances of the right atrial myxoma shown in Figure 136(b). (a) Tumor is associated with hemosiderin-containing phagocytes. (b) Atrial myxoma showing the typical benign tumor cells occurring in cords separated by interstitial space. (c) Variation in the histology of the myxoma is common. (d) Sparse, seemingly isolated tumor cells.

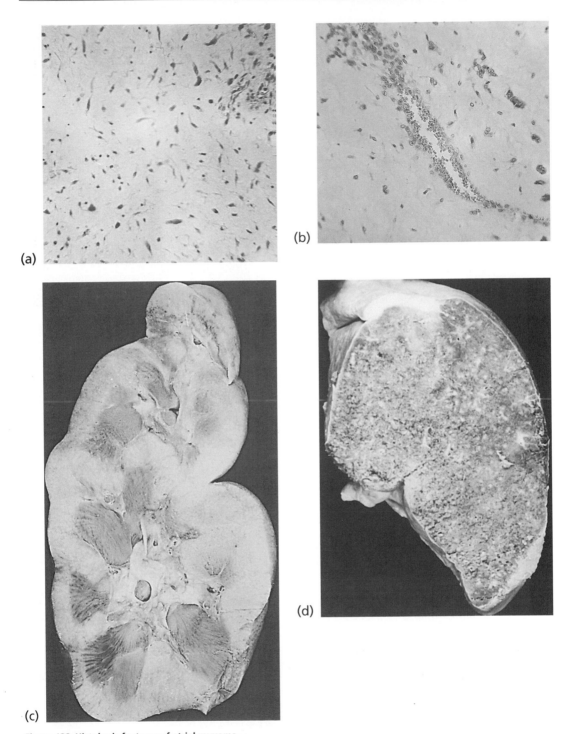

Figure 138 Histologic features of atrial myxoma.
(a,b) Histology of the atrial myxoma with spindle-shaped cells and a prominent interstitium. (c) Kidney with infarction due to embolic fragments of a left atrial myxoma. (d) Spleen with infarction due to embolic fragments of a left atrial myxoma.

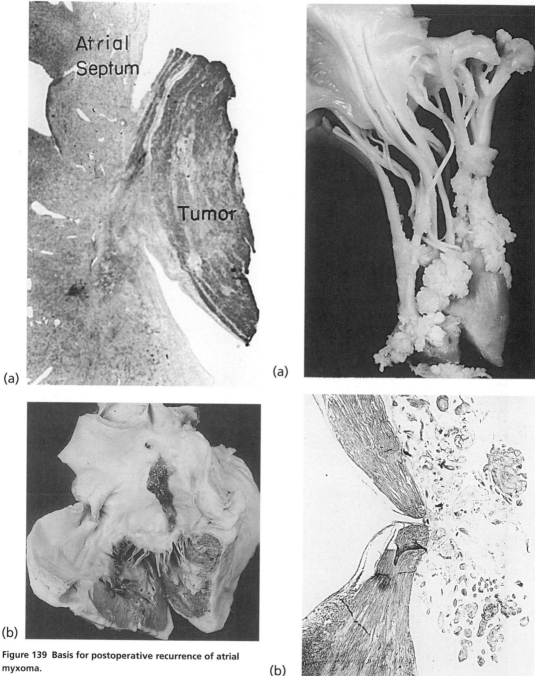

(a)

(a)

(b)

(b)

Figure 139 Basis for postoperative recurrence of atrial myxoma.
(a) Photomicrograph of the atrial septum including the stalk of a related left atrial myxoma. The stalk contains tumor and, if not removed, may cause recurrence. Male, 13 years. (b) Recurrent myxoma of the left atrium about 3 years postoperatively. Male, 68 years.

Figure 140 Papilloma of valves.
The papilloma may be seen starting in any of the valves. Obstruction may be caused by tumor protrusion into nearby chamber. Female, 62 years. (a) Surgically excised mitral valve with papillomas mostly attached to the chordae. The papillomas are benign. (b) Photomicrograph of a papilloma involving the tricuspid valve and right atrium.

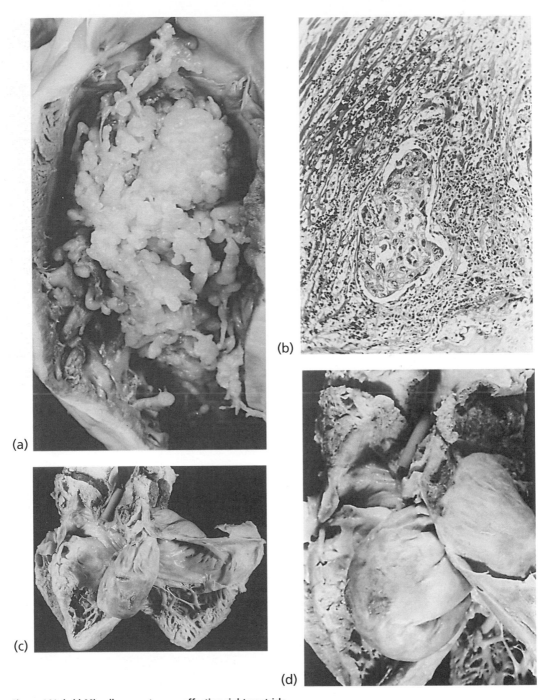

Figure 141 (a,b) Miscellaneous tumors affecting right ventricle.
(a) Teratoma of testis embolic to the right ventricle. The embolic mass was basically a testis with a tumor. It caused massive obstruction to filling of the right ventricle and sudden death. Male, 26 years. (b) Metastatic lesion in myocardium of choriocarcinoma. Female, 27 years.
(c,d) Thymoma with polypoid tumor invading the pulmonary artery and appearing in the right ventricle.
Right side of the heart with the tumor visualized. The tumor began in the thymus, invaded the pulmonary artery, and extended into the right ventricle and right atrium. Male, 15 years.

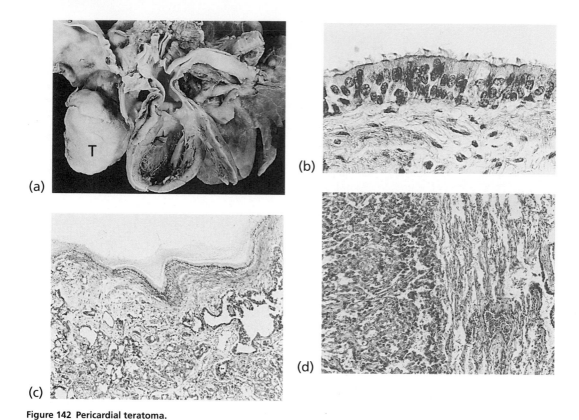

(a)

(b)

(c)

(d)

Figure 142 Pericardial teratoma.
Teratomas in the pericardial space area may affect children. As the name implies, many structures may occur within the tumor. Female, 2 years. (a) The heart and pericardial tissues with tumor (T) in the pericardium. (b) Photomicrograph of a portion of the pericardial teratoma with retinal tissue found within the tumor. (c,d) Photomicrographs of tumor tissue showing nonspecific vascular structure.

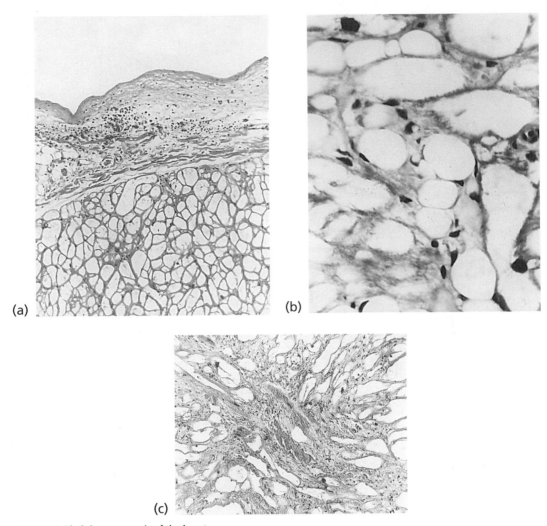
(a)
(b)
(c)

Figure 143 Rhabdomyomatosis of the heart.
(a) Infiltration of the myocardium by rhabdomyomatosis. A segment of myocardium with cells like those seen in rhabdomyomas but without distinct tumor nodules. (b) Higher power photomicrograph of conditions seen in (a). (c) Accumulations of giant cells in the myocardium, like those seen above.
Reprinted with permission from Shrivastava et al. [112].

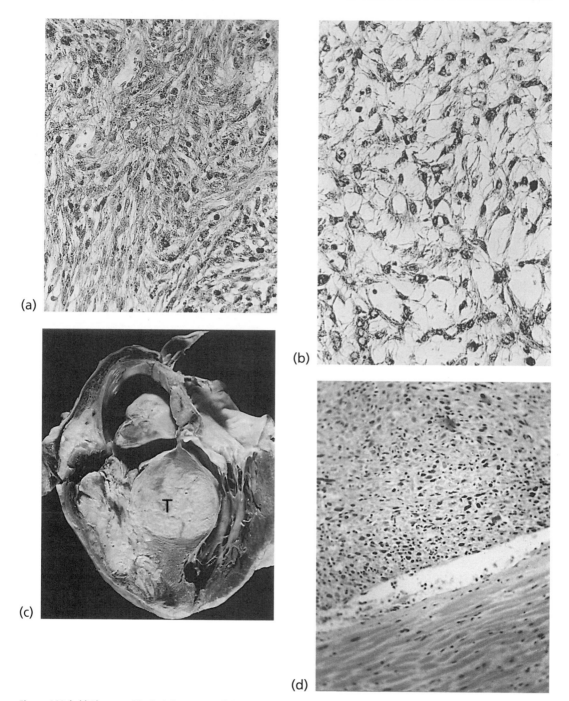

Figure 144 (a,b) Pleomorphic rhabdomyoma of the right ventricle.
Female, 14 years. (a,b) Photomicrographs of tumor formed by fusiform spindle cells.
(c,d) Sarcoma of the cardiac septa.
Female, 42 years. (c) Four-chamber view of the heart. There is a large tumor (T) within the ventricular septum and adjacent right ventricular wall, as well as a secondary mass adherent to the right atrial side of the atrial septum.
(d) Photomicrograph showing the tumor (above) involving the myocardium.

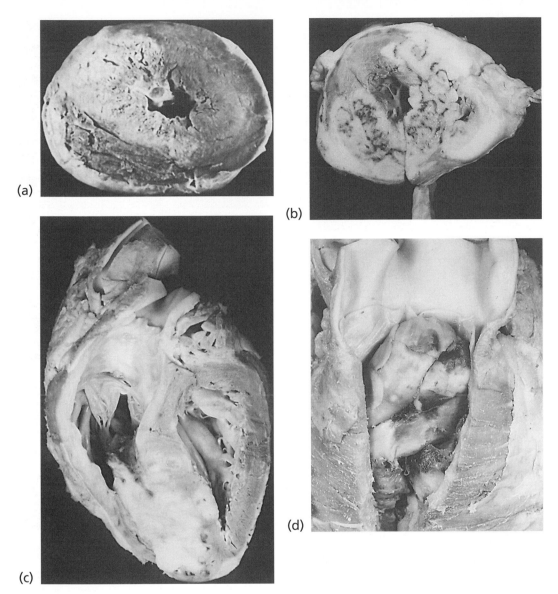

Figure 145 (a,b) Angiosarcoma of the ventricles.
(a) Tumor in adjacent parts of right and left ventricles and ventricular septum. Female, 40 years. (b) Tumor involving both ventricles with little preservation of normal myocardium.
(c,d) Metastatic myxosarcoma causing subpulmonary stenosis.
(c) The tumor involves the ventricular septum and right ventricle primarily. (d) A secondary tumor mass beneath the pulmonary valve causing major right ventricular outflow obstruction. Female, 22 years.

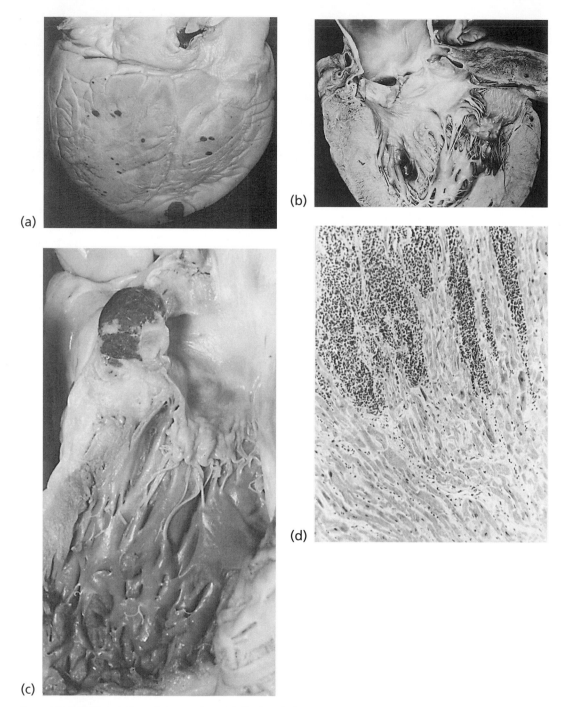

Figure 146 (a,b) Metastatic malignant melanoma affecting the heart.
Male, 53 years. (a) External view of the heart from behind. Metastatic melanoma (black dots) involving the epicardium.
(b) Tumor involving the endocardium and myocardium of the left ventricle.
(c,d) Malignant melanoma primary to the upper extremity metastatic to right atrium.
Male, 62 years. (c) Right atrium and ventricle. Metastatic tumor seen on the epicardial surface. (d) Histology of tumor
shown in (c) showing columns of invading melanoma.

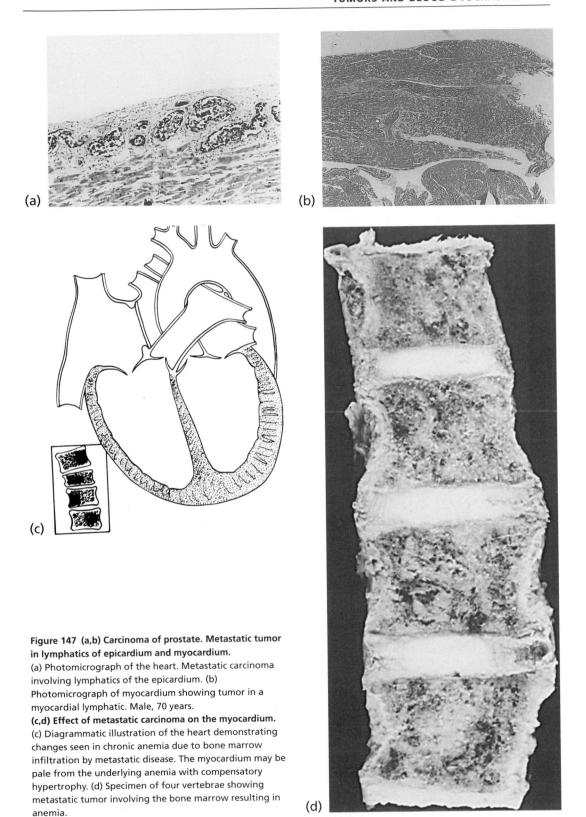

Figure 147 (a,b) Carcinoma of prostate. Metastatic tumor in lymphatics of epicardium and myocardium.
(a) Photomicrograph of the heart. Metastatic carcinoma involving lymphatics of the epicardium. (b) Photomicrograph of myocardium showing tumor in a myocardial lymphatic. Male, 70 years.
(c,d) Effect of metastatic carcinoma on the myocardium.
(c) Diagrammatic illustration of the heart demonstrating changes seen in chronic anemia due to bone marrow infiltration by metastatic disease. The myocardium may be pale from the underlying anemia with compensatory hypertrophy. (d) Specimen of four vertebrae showing metastatic tumor involving the bone marrow resulting in anemia.

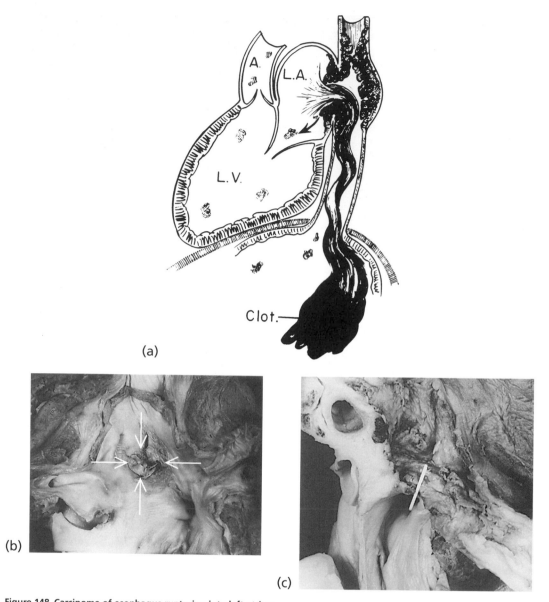

(a)

(b)

(c)

Figure 148 Carcinoma of esophagus rupturing into left atrium.
(a) Diagrammatic portrayal of carcinoma of esophagus eroding into left atrium and resulting in massive hemorrhage into the gastrointestinal tract. (b) Exterior of left atrium. Defect caused by invasion of left atrium by carcinoma of the esophagus (arrows). (c) Sagittal section through the esophagus and left atrium. The probe shows the path of continuity between the cavity of the left atrium and the lumen of the esophagus.
Reprinted with permission from Edwards [109].

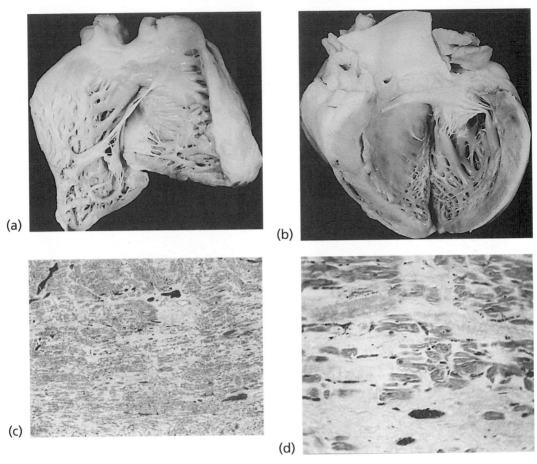

Figure 149 Myocardial failure from administration of Adriamycin.
Male, 17 years. (a) Interior right ventricle. The chamber is dilated secondary to congestive heart failure. (b) Dilatation of the left ventricle in a patient who received Adriamycin. Grossly the heart affected by Adriamycin is indistinguishable from that with a dilated cardiomyopathy. (c,d) Each photomicrograph shows effects of Adriamycin. In each illustration there is loss of continuity in the myocardial fibers.

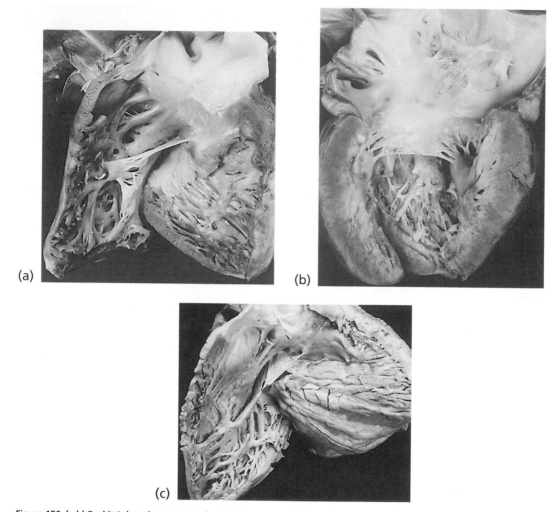

(a)

(b)

(c)

Figure 150 (a,b) Burkitt's lymphoma treated with Cytoxan and Adriamycin; myocardial hemorrhages.
Male, 6 years. (a) Interior right ventricle. The chamber is dilated. The endocardium is thickened. There is hemorrhage at the apex. (b) The left ventricle shows endocardial fibroelastosis.
(c) Right ventricle dilation in leukemia treated with chemotherapy.
Female, 39 years. (c) The right ventricle is dilated; this may be a consequence of chemotherapy or the response to chronic anemia.

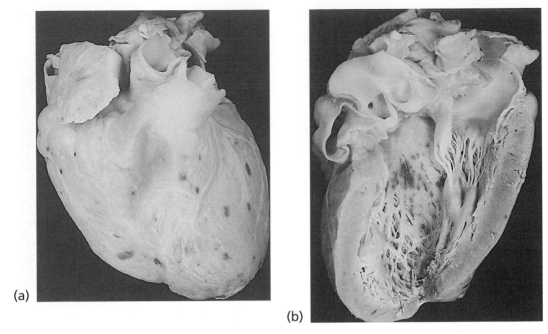

(a)

(b)

Figure 151 Blood dyscrasia associated with cardiac disorders.
Aplastic anemia with thrombocytopenia. (a) Exterior of heart showing multiple epicardial hemorrhages. (b) Left side of heart showing hemorrhage into the myocardium. Female, 6 years.

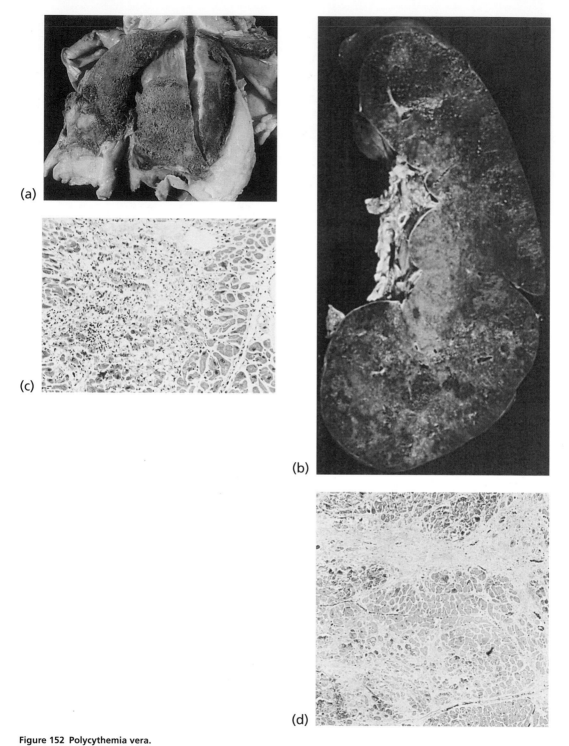

Figure 152 Polycythemia vera.
(a) External view of the heart and pericardium. There is diffuse pericardial hemorrhage. (b) Spleen showing marked enlargement. (c,d) Photomicrographs of myocardium showing hemorrhages and scarring.

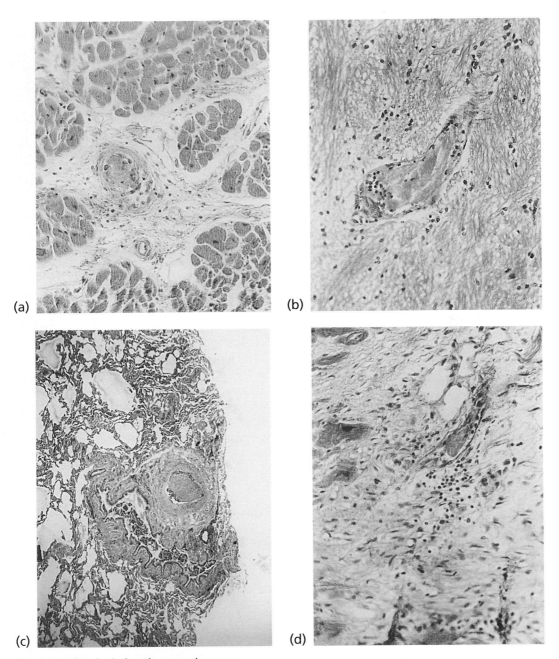

(a)

(b)

(c)

(d)

Figure 153 Thrombotic thrombocytopenic purpura.
(a) Myocardium showing interstitial hemorrhage and thrombus in an arteriole. Male, 43 years. (b) A second case with thrombus in the intramyocardial small artery. Male, 40 years. (c) Lung with a thrombus in an arteriole. Male, 40 years. (d) Myocardium shows small focal scars and a mild cellular infiltrate. Male, 40 years.

CHAPTER 9

Great vessels and related structures

Superior and inferior vena cavae

This section considers the superior vena cava and inferior vena cava as relates to intrinsic diseases of these structures. The cavae may be the sites of venous thrombosis leading to pulmonary embolism and the development of secondary pulmonary hypertension.

The left-sided systemic veins are longer than the right-sided veins; thus, in general, left-sided veins are more susceptible to thrombosis than right-sided veins. The superior vena cava is less likely to be subject to thrombosis than the inferior vena cava. Superior vena caval thromboses are more apt to be significant depending on the position of the thrombus relative to the entrance of the azygos vein. Because of the potential for collateral flow when the azygos vein lies superior to the obstruction, the venous obstruction is less significant than when the obstruction is inferior to the azygos vein.

In general, the superior vena cava is resistant to thrombosis except in the presence of malignant tumors, especially carcinoma of the lung and lymphomas or by the presence of chronic indwelling catheters or device leads.

The inferior vena cava is very susceptible to thrombosis, even during bedrest for minor illnesses. Given a background of immobility due to a serious disease, such as acute myocardial infarction or surgical treatment of a tumor, thrombosis of the ileofemoral system is a significant risk. Once ileofemoral thrombosis occurs, healing may be complicated by destruction of venous valves resulting in venous incompetence and the likelihood of further thrombosis [113].

Renal cell carcinoma, with extension of tumor into the renal vein, may extend further into the inferior vena cava yielding a potential for pulmonary tumor embolism [114].

The integrity of the atrial septum may have great significance for patients who develop venous thrombosis. The foramen ovale is located in the right side of the atrial septum. From this is a channel that leads through the atrial septum and enters the left atrium at the interatrial ostium II; this channel is vital in the fetus as it carries oxygenated blood originating from the placenta to the left side of the heart. Usually, the channel closes shortly after birth. However in about 30% of people. A patent foramen ovale (PFO) remains. The Valsalva maneuver (whether done intentionally or unintentionally such as on a roller coaster ride) may make a potential communication a real communication between the atria. If the opening from the right atrium to the left atrium is persistent after birth, an embolus may cross the atrial septum from right to left as a paradoxical embolus. Both atrial septal aneurysm and patent foramen ovale are risk factors for cryptogenic stroke [115]. PFO with right to left shunting may represent a risk factor for recurrent migraine heatachos [116].

Pulmonary hypertension

All types of pulmonary hypertension may be associated with syncope and sudden death. Pulmonary hypertension may be divided into primary and secondary types. The more common entity, secondary pulmonary hypertension, will be presented first.

Secondary pulmonary hypertension

Secondary pulmonary hypertension occurs as the result of many conditions, including pulmonary embolism, fibrotic lung disease, thoracic skeletal deformities, and obesity. Regardless of the cause, right ventricular hypertrophy is universally present in chronic states of pulmonary hypertension.

Pulmonary embolism is a major cause of secondary pulmonary hypertension. Pulmonary emboli vary in appearance and age; their shape is affected by the sites of formation. Fresh emboli may be associated with pulmonary infarcts. Old emboli may undergo organization with replacement of connective tissue forming in the pulmonary arteries [117]. Patients with pulmonary hypertension due to recurrent emboli may improve after surgical removal of the organized clot and associated fibrotic material.

Pulmonary hypertension may occur secondary to diseases of the lung. Among these causes are parenchymal pulmonary diseases including emphysema, chronic obstructive pulmonary disease, fibrotic lung disease, and cystic fibrosis. Other causes of secondary pulmonary hypertension include obesity, sleep apnea, embolism of tumor to the pulmonary vasculature, fat embolism, and amniotic embolism. We have even observed pulmonary embolism of hepatic tissue resulting from an explosion. Pulmonary embolism may complicate gastric bypass surgery [118].

Fat embolism

Fat embolism is usually made up of neutral fat. Classically, fat embolism is one of the observed complications from long bone fractures. In modern times fat embolism may be seen as a complication of surgical treatment of the hip and/or the knee. Basically, the lesion starts from injury to the bone and the fat travels in the peripheral venous system through the right side of the heart to the lung. If a patent foramen ovale is present, the fat embolus may cross from the right atrium into the left atrium affecting the systemic circulation. For patients with a large patent foramen ovale (PFO) and right-to-left shunting, it has been suggested that one consider device closure of the PFO before elective surgical manipulation of the hip or knee. This could have important protective effects against massive systemic fat embolization.

According to Pitto et al., intraoperative prophylaxis against fat and bone marrow embolism during total hip arthroplasty can reduce the incidence of postoperative deep vein thrombosis [119].

Primary pulmonary hypertension

Primary pulmonary hypertension is commonly divided into three pathologic types: the plexogenic type, the thromboembolic type, and veno-occlusive disease. In each condition there is hypertrophy of the right ventricle and the media of the pulmonary arterial vessels. In the plexogenic type there is remodeling of the pulmonary vasculature with formation of plexogenic lesions [120]. In the thromboembolic type the arterial vessels are occluded by thrombotic material; this may occur in large or medium-sized arteries. In veno-occlusive disease the primary site of obstruction to flow is at the pulmonary veins and venules. In the veno-occlusive form [121], cardiac catheterization usually does not show an elevation of pulmonary capillary wedge pressure despite the fact that the primary lesion is postcapillary.

Coexistent pulmonary hypertension and portal hypertension

Patients with portal hypertension of varying etiology may develop pulmonary arterial hypertension. Edwards and associates [122] reported on the subject of coexisting pulmonary and portal hypertension. Plexogenic pulmonary arteriopathy was present in 10 patients, seven of whom also had coexistent thromboembolic lesions.

Pulmonary arterial aneurysm

Butto and associates [123] described vessels in which noninflammatory pulmonary arterial aneurysmal disease existed. In each case, severe pulmonary hypertension had been present. In one woman, aged 50 years, the pulmonary hypertension was of the primary type; in each of the others, congenital heart disease was an underlying condition. Cystic medial necrosis was present and the aneurysmal disease was the result of spontaneous laceration of a pulmonary arterial segment.

Diseases of the aorta

The following selected aortic subjects, which can present with sudden death, will be discussed in this section: traumatic lesions; systemic arterial occlusion; atherosclerotic lesions, including aneurysms; aortitis; aortic dissection; and aortic- or arterial-esophageal fistula.

Traumatic lesions of the aorta

Lesions of the aorta resulting from trauma tend to be localized in three sites, namely the ascending aorta [124] (leading to hemopericardium), the descending aorta at the level of the ligamentum arteriosum (leading to left hemothorax), and the junction of the right subclavian artery from the in nominante artery. The ductus arteriosus (right or left) provides a point of fixation for the aorta. With deceleration injuries there may be torsion of the aorta around the ductus leading to a tear; this would result in a tear adjacent to the innominate artery in the presence of a right ductus, or a tear of the descending aorta in the presence of a left ductus.

Systemic arterial occlusion

Systemic arterial occlusion, in general, tends to affect either major arteries or small arteries. Arterial occlusion may be caused by primary arterial disease, including atherosclerosis, arteritis, and primary thrombotic disorders, or by systemic embolism.

Atherosclerotic lesions

Atherosclerotic lesions have a tendency for a wide variety of complications. Localized atherosclerotic lesions may be the source of thrombosis, embolism, and localized stenosis, particularly in the aorta and coronary, femoral, and cerebral arteries.

Aneurysm formation

Atherosclerosis has a tendency to form aneurysms, particularly in the abdominal aorta but also affecting other peripheral vessels. Aneurysms of the abdominal aorta, classically, lie inferior to the origin of the renal arteries and superior to the bifurcation of the aorta. The inferior mesenteric artery frequently arises from the aneurysmal part of the abdominal aorta. In some cases, despite the aneurysm, the artery remains patent; otherwise it may be occluded by atherosclerosis or thrombus. The major complication of abdominal aortic aneurysm is rupture. The abdominal aorta lies in close proximity to the third portion of the duodenum; rarely, a ruptured abdominal aortic aneurysm is directed into the duodenum. While the inferior vena cava lies in close relationship to the abdominal aorta, it is rare that rupture of the aorta would lead into the nearby inferior vena cava. In a case demonstrated in this book, an aneurysm of the abdominal aorta did rupture into the inferior vena cava creating a massive arterial-venous fistula with the interesting occurrence of cholesterol emboli in the pulmonary arterial system. Infection may occur in abdominal aortic aneurysm. This phenomenon may lead to major complications including rupture as well as various arterial occlusions.

Aortitis

The distribution of inflammatory lesions in aortitis may involve the aorta itself or the combination of the aorta and the pulmonary artery. The etiology and manifestations of aortitis can be categorized as bacterial aortitis, fungal aortitis, syphilitic aortitis, tuberculous aortitis, and a group of inflammatory diseases of the aorta that may include Takayasu aortitis.

Various organisms, including *Salmonella*, may cause bacterial aortitis, affecting the aorta and its branches. Bacterial aortitis may be associated with infection of one or more cardiac valves. The aortic lesion is highly destructive and may be associated with infectious vasculitis of the aorta or of various branches of the aorta [125]. Fungal aortitis, which is rare in immunocompetent hosts, may be caused by *Aspergillus* species. This can be seen after aortic or coronary surgery [126]. The condition of syphilitic aortitis is now a rare entity among areas that aggressively treat infectious diseases. Syphilitic aortitis affects the thoracic aorta with medial inflammatory disease, calcification, and secondary atherosclerosis; the coronary arterial ostia may be narrowed. Tuberculous aortitis is a condition that is rare in the United States. According to Choi and associates [127] tuberculous aortitis generally develops in the distal aortic arch and the descending aorta. These authors reported a case of tuberculous aortitis with rupture of the ascending aorta. In cases of aortitis the aortic valve cusps may be distorted, allowing for aortic regurgitation. Takayasu aortitis [128] is most frequently reported in the Asian population (although it occurs internationally) and affects young women far more often than men. The histology of the lesions in Takayasu aortitis varies considerably from case to case. Included in the histologic pictures are such features as atrophy of the media, interstitial leukocytic infiltration, giant cell infiltration, and areas of fibrosis. In some cases of Takayasu aortitis the pulmonary trunk is simultaneously involved.

Temporal arteritis and aortitis

The syndrome of temporal arteritis and aortitis is a classic subject [129]. In temporal arteritis, the inflammatory infiltrate includes giant cells. A variation may be characterized by atypical infiltrates or nongranulomatous arteritis. Healed temporal arteritis is characterized by intimal fibrosis and medial scarring with segmental disruption of the internal elastic lamina. Atypical giant cell arteritis shows occlusive intimal fibrosis with diffuse granulomatous inflammation of the media. Temporal arteritis may be associated with the syndrome of temporomandibular pain, visual changes and jaw claudication.

Aortic dissection

The etiologies of aortic dissection vary widely. Hypertension is a common precursor. Hypertension and coarctation together increase the likelihood of aortic dissection. Atherosclerosis is an uncommon basis for this condition. Cystic medial necrosis [130] is commonly seen in aortic dissection, associated with either arachnodactyly (Marfan syndrome) or bicuspid aortic valve, aortic stenosis, and myxomatous mitral valve.

Aortic dissection starts as a break in the intima of the aorta; through the break, a tract (false passage) develops into the media. The length of the tract in the media varies and usually ends by "re-rupturing" through the intima into the lumen of the aorta creating the "double barreled aorta." If the dissection track extends not back into the lumen but to the adventitia, rapid exsanguination typically occurs. There are three types of dissection that are recognized: In type I, the false tract runs the length of the aorta from the ascending aorta into one of the iliac arteries. In type II, the dissection starts above the coronary origins and ends at the origins of the branches of the aortic arch. The third type begins beyond the left subclavian artery and descends for varying distances down the descending aorta. As the false passage extends, the affected branches may be significantly obstructed; classical sites of obstruction may include coronary arteries, carotid arteries, and the left renal artery. The left renal artery is affected due to the location of the dissection on the left side of the abdominal aorta, which compresses the left renal artery; the phenomenon is frequently associated with infarction of the left kidney. The right-sided segmental spinal arteries are rarely affected, even in cases of extensive aortic dissection. There is infarction of the spinal cord only in rare cases because of the maintenance of blood flow through the right-sided spinal arteries.

Aortic- or arterial-esophageal fistula

A false passage between the aorta and esophagus may develop easily because of their close proximity to each other. The fistula may develop from an aortic aneurysm, esophageal diverticula, foreign bodies in the esophagus, or esophageal neoplasm. The erosion may lead to an initially minor gastrointestinal (GI) hemorrhage, known as a "sentinel" hemorrhage, before developing into massive GI bleeding [131].

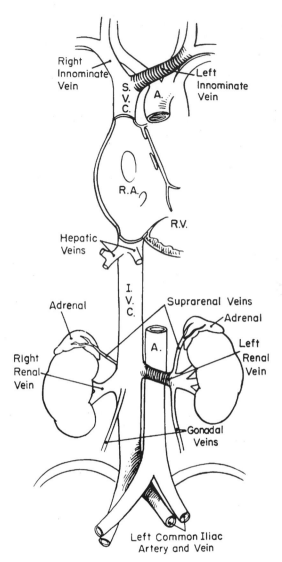

Figure 154 Systemic veins.
Drawing of major systemic veins. Cross-hatched veins are left sided indicating the greater length than right-sided veins.
Theoretically, the left-sided veins tend to be more susceptible to thrombosis.

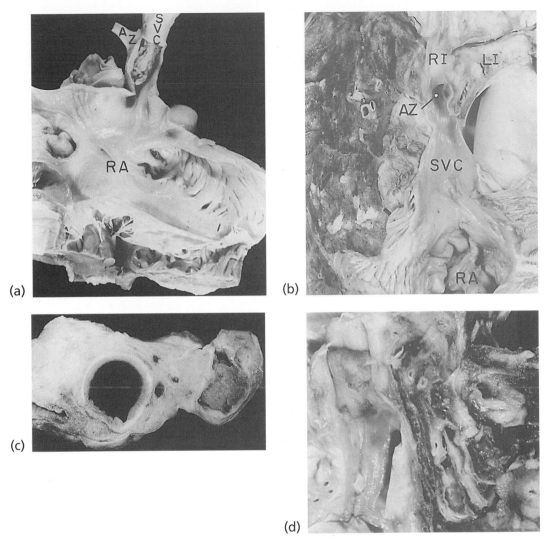

Figure 155 Superior vena cava and the azygos vein.
(a) Superior vena cava (SVC) containing thrombus, joining right atrium. Position of azygous vein (AZ) is shown. Male, 59 years. (b) Superior vena cava formed by right innominate (RI) and left innominate (LI) veins and joining right atrium (RA). AZ, azygos vein. Male, 73 years. (c) Cross section of the upper mediastinal structures. Mediastinal lymphoma surrounding trachea and part of the esophagus. Superior vena cava at right containing thrombus. Female, 51 years. (d) Thrombus of superior vena cava. Background tissues contain metastatic tumors from bronchogenic carcinoma.

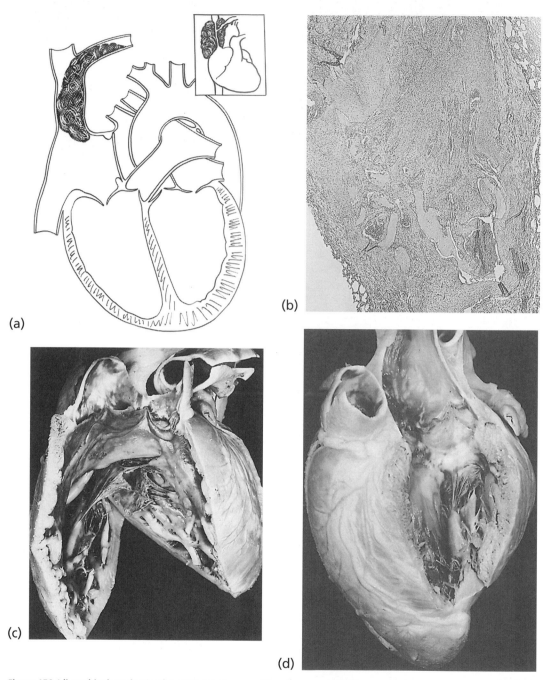

Figure 156 Idiopathic thrombosis of superior vena cava with pulmonary emboli.
(a) Diagrammatic portrayal of thrombus in superior vena cava. Insert shows tumor surrounding superior vena cava not present in this case. (b) Photomicrograph of thrombus in superior vena cava. (c) Right ventricle showing hypertrophy due to pulmonary hypertension, in this case caused by recurrent thromboembolism in the lungs. (d) Left ventricle normal. Female, 32 years.

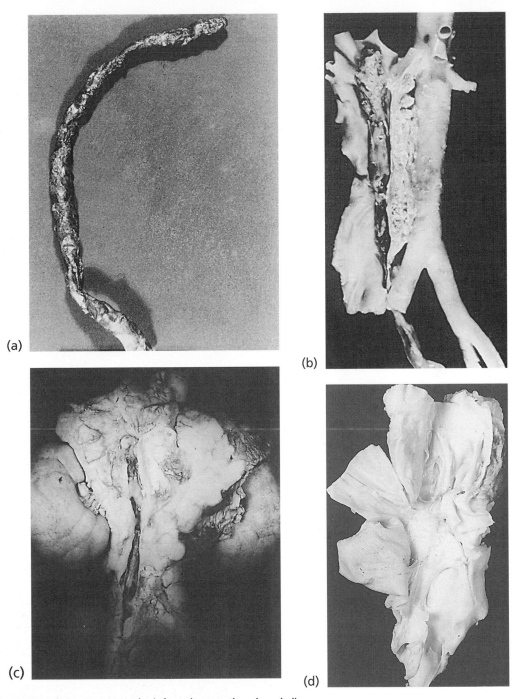

Figure 157 Inferior vena cava; a basis for pulmonary thromboembolism.
Thrombosis of the inferior vena cava is vastly more susceptible to pulmonary embolism than thrombosis of the superior vena cava. In many patients thrombosis occurs without malignant disease. (a) Large thrombosis extracted from right and left kidneys, femoral venous system. (b) Abdominal aorta and inferior vena cava. The latter contains a thrombus as a potential for pulmonary embolism. There is no evidence for external compression of the vena cava or aorta. Male, 61 years. (c) Inferior vena cava with thrombus. The vein is surrounded by metastatic malignant tissue. (d) Segment of inferior vena cava showing an organized thrombus. At this stage, the thrombus has partially recanalized. Male, 57 years. Reprinted with permission from Edwards [55].

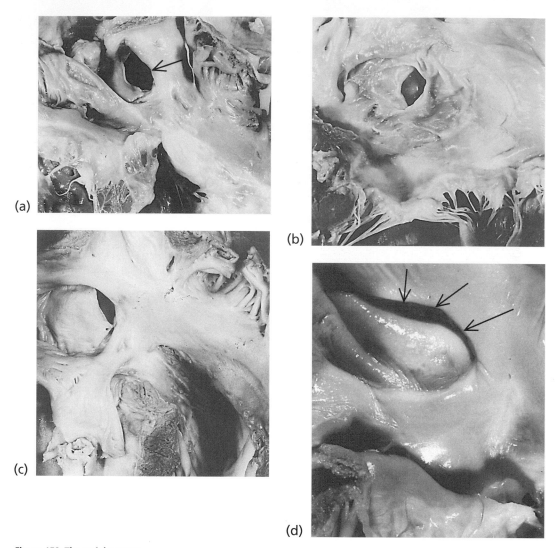

(a)

(b)

(c)

(d)

Figure 158 The atrial septum.
Patent foramen ovale and aneurysm of foramen ovale. (a) Right atrium showing a small atrial septal defect (arrow).
(b) Left atrium showing a small atrial septal defect. (c) Shortening of the valve of a patent foramen ovale allows for flow
of blood in either direction. Female, 2 days. (d) Foramen ovale. The crescent-shaped dark shadow (arrows) is a thrombus
in a valvular competent foramen ovale. The thrombus has the potential for either pulmonary or systemic embolism. Male,
56 years.

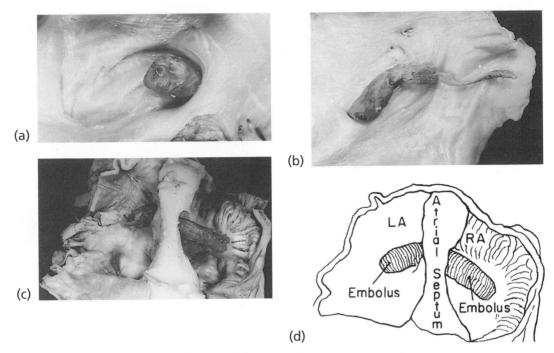

Figure 159 Classical paradoxical embolism through foramen ovale.
(a) Right atrial opening of a patent foramen ovale showing the tail of a paradoxical embolus. (b) Left atrium showing the head of a paradoxical embolus. Male, 74 years. (c) A second case of paradoxical embolus. The atrial septum has been sectioned so that the paradoxical embolus is seen from both sides, as shown diagrammatically in (d).

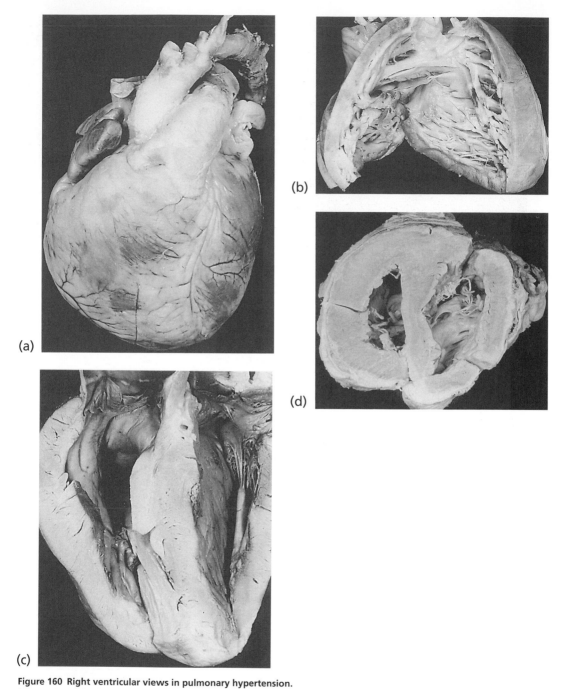

(a)

(b)

(c)

(d)

Figure 160 Right ventricular views in pulmonary hypertension.
(a) Exterior of the heart showing prominence of the area of the right ventricle and pulmonary artery. Female, 8 years.
(b) Massive right ventricular hypertrophy. (c) Interior of the ventricles from the front. The ventricular septum is central
and hypertrophied. The right ventricle is on the left and hypertrophied. The left ventricle is shown for comparison.
(d) Ventricles shown in cross section and viewed from below. The right ventricle (right side of illustration) is
hypertrophied. The left ventricle is also hypertrophied. There is classic flattening of the ventricular septum forming the
"D"-shaped septum.

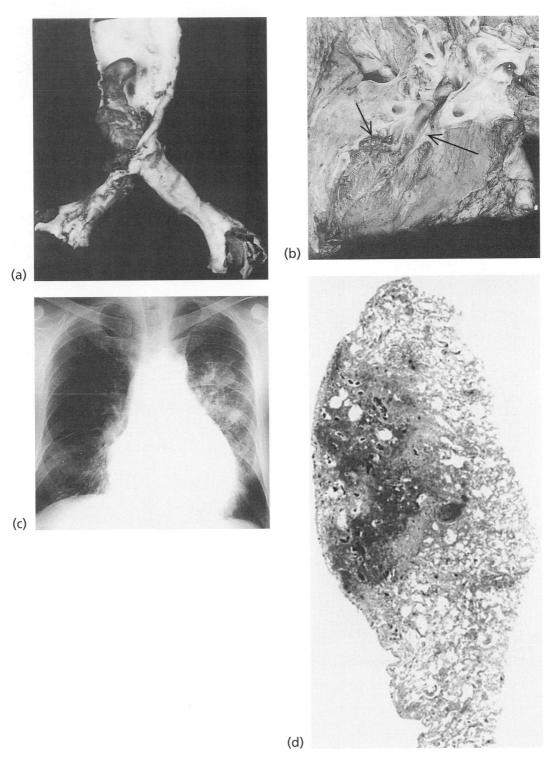

Figure 161 Classical case of pulmonary embolism.
(a) Inferior vena cava and iliac veins containing thrombi. (b) Lung showing pulmonary emboli (arrows). (c) Radiograph of the thorax. Pulmonary infarction of the left lower lobe. (d) Segment of left lung showing recent pulmonary infarcts.

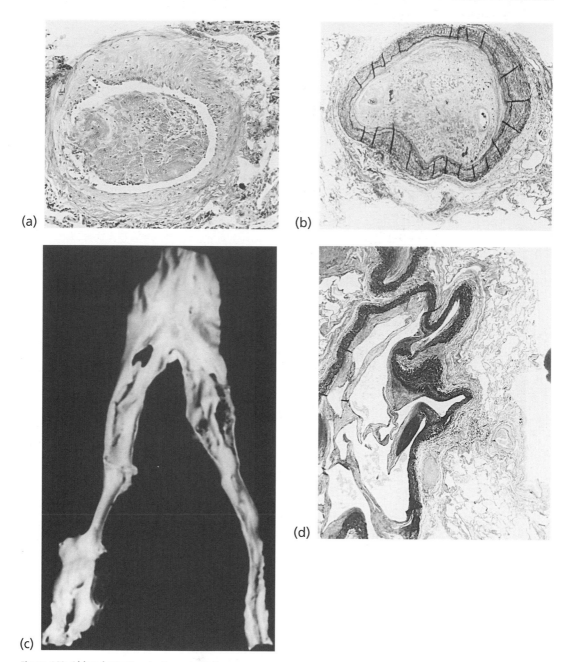

Figure 162 Old and recent pulmonary emboli.
(a) Photomicrograph of pulmonary artery emboli about 2 days old. (b) Emboli about 1 week old. Female, 67 years.
(c) Inferior vena cava and iliac veins. Partially recanalized thrombi. (d) Pulmonary artery contains remnants of organized thrombi. Female, 57 years.

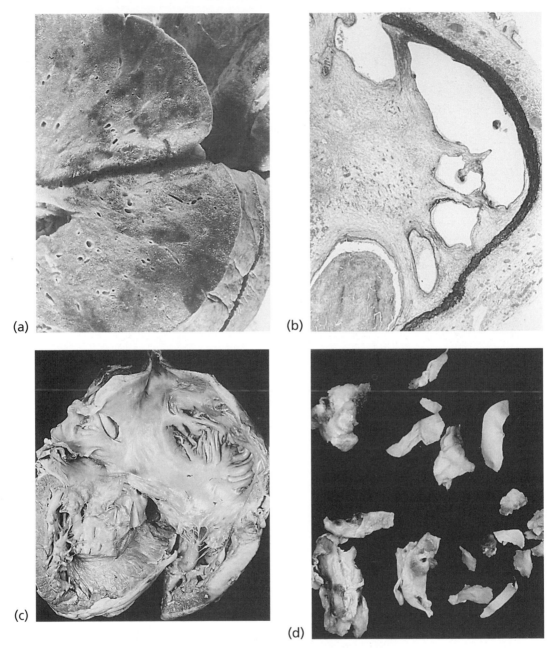

(a)

(b)

(c)

(d)

Figure 163 (a,b) Chronic pulmonary emboli of different ages.
(a) Gross specimen of lung. Multiple pulmonary infarcts. Male, 34 years. (b) High power photomicrograph of pulmonary artery showing thrombosis with partial recanalization. Sudden death. Male, 32 years.
(c,d) Chronic pulmonary emboli, resected surgically; early postoperative death.
Female, 58 years. (c) Right side of heart with right ventricular hypertrophy. (d) Specimens resected during pulmonary thromboendartectomy consisting of organized thrombus.

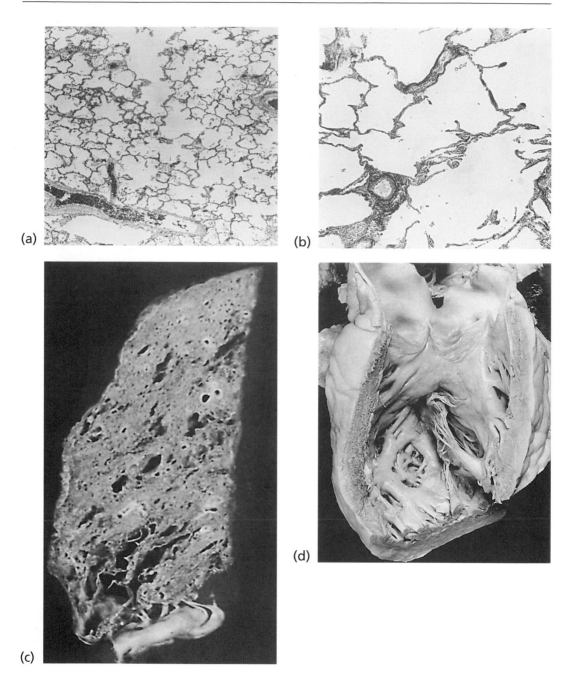

Figure 164 Secondary causes of pulmonary hypertension: emphysema.
(a) Photomicrograph. Normal tissue of lung for comparison. (b) Photomicrograph of lung. Pulmonary emphysema with loss of alveolar septa. (c) Gross specimen of lung. Pulmonary fibrosis with cavitation. (d) Right ventricular hypertrophy in secondary pulmonary hypertension. Female, 60 years.

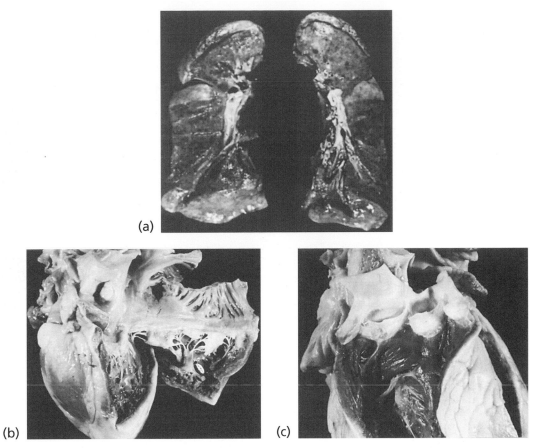

(a)

(b)   (c)

Figure 165 Pulmonary fibrosis causing pulmonary hypertension.
(a) The lungs showing diffuse pulmonary fibrosis. (b) Right ventricle and tricuspid valve. Right ventricular hypertrophy.
(c) Pulmonary artery and right ventricle. Right ventricular hypertrophy.

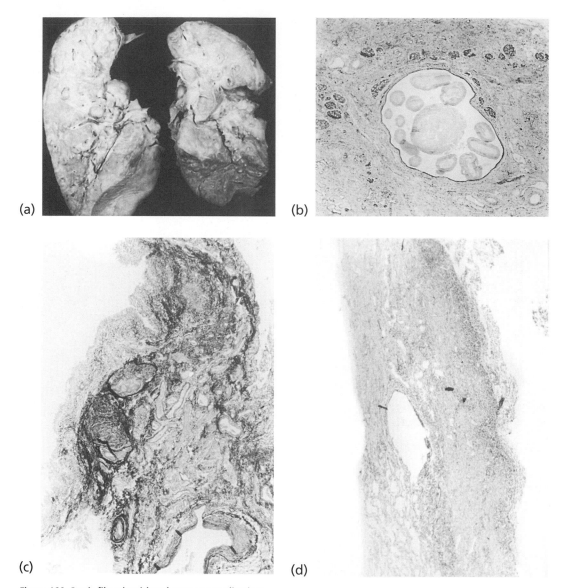

Figure 166 Cystic fibrosis with pulmonary complications.
Female, 19 years. (a) Gross specimen of the lung from young woman with cystic fibrosis. (b) Chronic inflammation of the lung. Foreign body aspertion within bronchus. (c) Photomicrograph of lung. Chronic abscess secondary to cystic fibrosis. (d) Segment of collapsed lung.

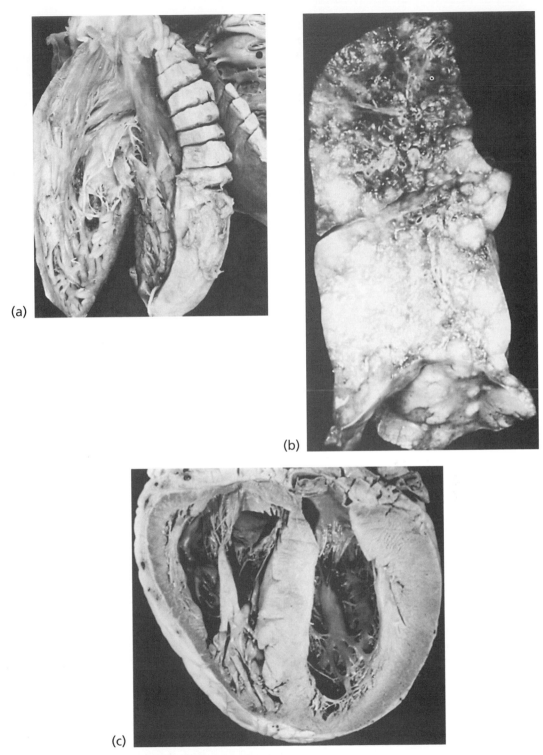

Figure 167 Miscellaneous causes of pulmonary hypertension.
(a) Right ventricle in a patient with kyphoscoliosis and restrictive pulmonary disease. There is right ventricular hypertrophy. Female, 37 years. (b) Lung. Extensive replacement by tumor causing reduction in the normal pulmonary vascular bed and secondary pulmonary hypertension. (c) Obstructive sleep apnea (Pickwick's syndrome): ventricular chambers showing right ventricular hypertrophy. Section of both ventricles. Male, 33 years.

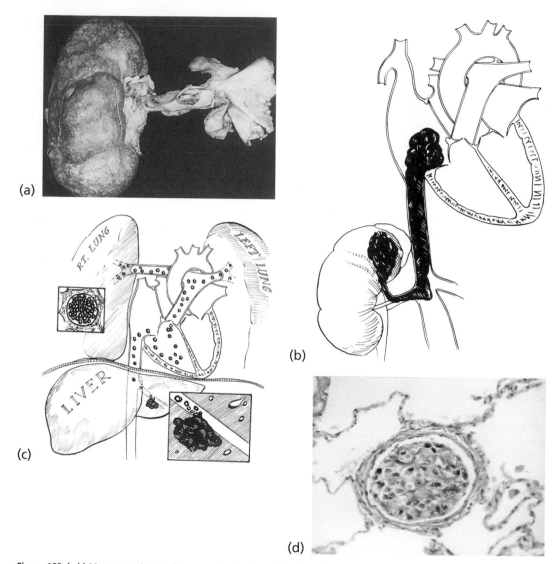

Figure 168 (a,b) Metastases into pulmonary arteries through major veins.
(a) Kidney and renal vein. Tumor of kidney extending into the renal vein. (b) Diagrammatic portrayal of the phenomenon shown in (a). The tumor may extend directly into the right-sided cardiac chambers and even the pulmonary artery. In the later case, the tumor hemodynamically, may be equivalent to a pulmonary embolism.
(c,d) Metastases into pulmonary arteries of microscopic size.
(c) Diagrammatic portrayal of process of embolism to microscopic-sized pulmonary arteries from a hepatic tumor. (d) Photomicrograph of small pulmonary artery containing metastatic tumor.

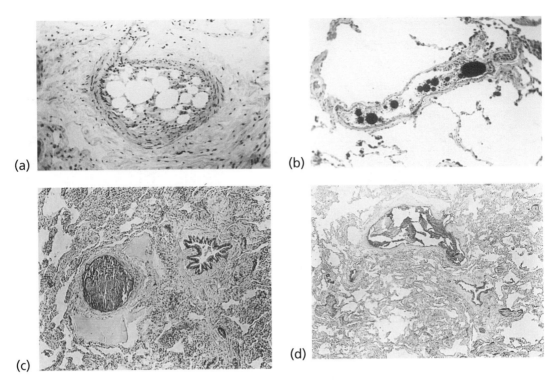

(a)

(b)

(c)

(d)

Figure 169 (a,b) Fat embolism.
Multiple factors and injuries involving soft tissues may give rise to fat embolism, which is characterized by neutral fat in the small arteries and arterioles in the body. (a) Small systemic arteriole containing fat cells. (b) Fat embolism to the lung. Tissue stained for fat reveals dark particles of fat in the lumen.

(c,d) Amniotic pulmonary embolism.
In the late stages of labor and in the setting of a difficult delivery, sudden death may occur in the mother. The condition may be caused by amniotic embolism into the pulmonary arteries. (c,d) Pulmonary tissues revealing presence of amniotic fluid within smaller arterial vessels. Female, 45 years.

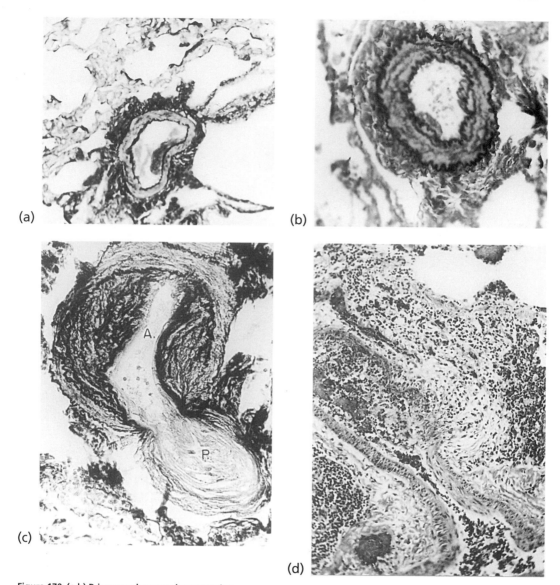

Figure 170 (a,b) Primary pulmonary hypertension.
(a) A normal pulmonary artery. Female, 34 years. (b) Medial hypertrophy of a pulmonary artery. Female, 22 months.
(c,d) Primary pulmonary hypertension: plexogenic type.
Female, 4 years. (c) A pulmonary artery showing plexogenic deformity. A, artery; P, plexiform lesion. (d) Medial
hypertrophy and distruction of arterial wall in a pulmonary artery associated with acute inflammation.
Reprinted with permission from Edwards and Edwards [175].

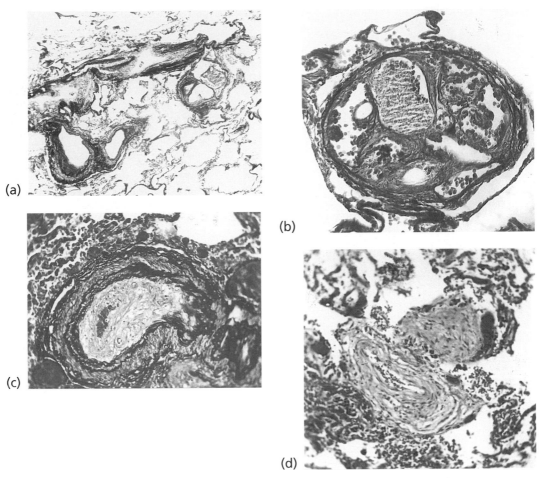

Figure 171 (a,b) Primary pulmonary hypertension: thromboembolic type.
Male, 56 years. (a) Medial hypertrophy of the muscular arteries and formations of organized thrombi. (b) A pulmonary artery showing organized thrombus and medial hypertrophy. There is evidence of recanalization.
Reprinted with permission from Edwards and Edwards [175].
(c,d) Cirrhosis of liver with pulmonary hypertension.
(c) Photomicrograph of pulmonary artery showing medial hypertrophy and organized thrombus in pulmonary artery from a patient with cirrhosis of the liver. (d) A small pulmonary artery showing major intimal proliferation.

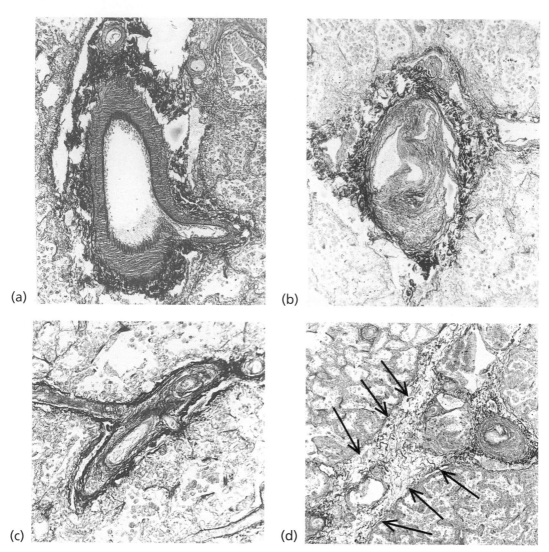

(a)

(b)

(c)

(d)

Figure 172 Primary pulmonary hypertension: pulmonary veno-occlusive disease.
Female, 4 years. Photomicrographs. (a) A small pulmonary artery with medial hypertrophy. (b) A small pulmonary vein obstructed by an organized thrombus. (c) Pulmonary vein showing intimal fibrosis. (d) Lymphatic (between arrows) showing dilatation as a sign of elevated pulmonary capillary pressure.
Reprinted with permission from Anderson et al. [121].

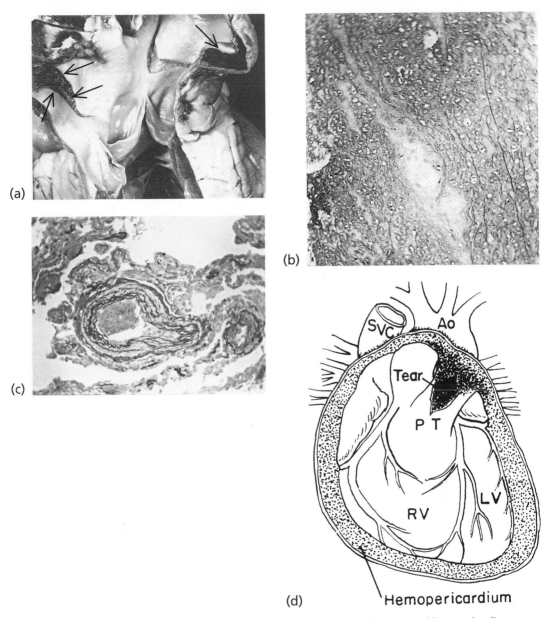

Figure 173 Complication of chronic pulmonary hypertension: pulmonary arterial dissection and hemopericardium.
Sudden death. Female, 63 years. (a) Pulmonary artery showing a major tear (arrows) just above the pulmonary valve.
(b) Photomicrograph of pulmonary artery showing cystic medial necrosis, secondary to long-standing pulmonary
hypertension. (c) Photomicrograph of small pulmonary artery showing medial hypertrophy as a sign of pulmonary
hypertension. (d) Diagram demonstrating a tear in pulmonary trunk resulting in hemopericardium and sudden death.

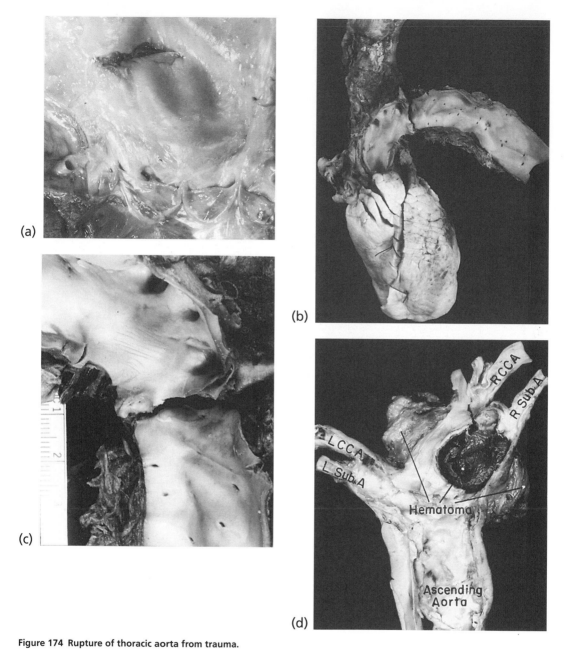

(a)

(b)

(c)

(d)

Figure 174 Rupture of thoracic aorta from trauma.
(a) Primary laceration of ascending aorta above the aortic valve. Male, 86 years. (b) Laceration of descending thoracic aorta with massive hemorrhage. Male, 68 years. (c) Interior view of the aorta. Laceration of descending aorta at the level of ligamentum arteriosum following thoracic trauma. Hemorrhage into the left pleural space. Male, 19 years. In the rare circumstances where a patient may survive this type of tear, a chronic posttraumatic aneurysm will develop at this site. (d) Ascending aorta and aortic arch; view from behind. A major hematoma is present at the root of the innominate artery.

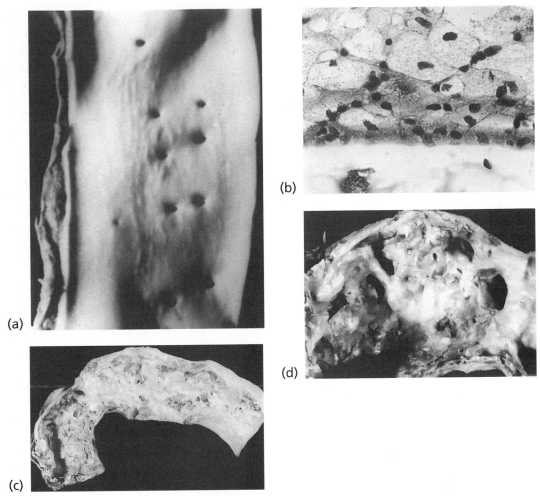

Figure 175 Atherosclerosis of the aorta: from beginning to end.
(a) Gross photograph of opened thoracic aorta. Beside the ostia of the intercostal arteries are yellow elevations, called "fatty streaks," said to be among the earliest of atherosclerotic lesions. (b) Photomicrograph of an aorta demonstrating fatty streaks. (c,d) Segments of the aorta in a person with end-stage aortic atherosclerotic disease. The lumen is ulcerated and friable.

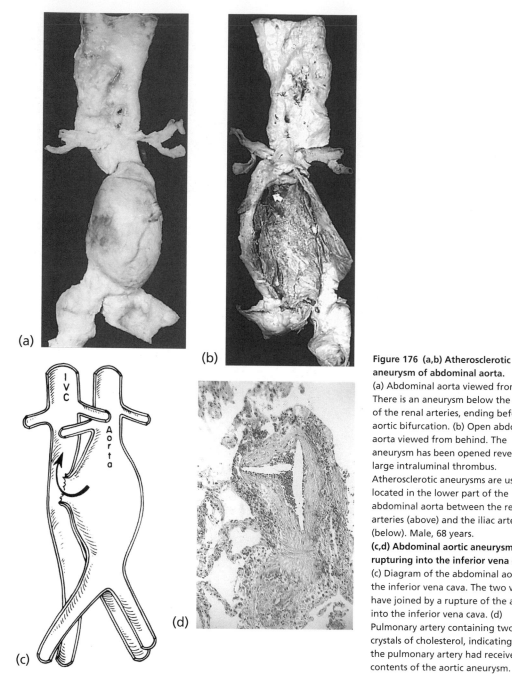

(a)

(b)

(c)

(d)

Figure 176 (a,b) Atherosclerotic aneurysm of abdominal aorta.
(a) Abdominal aorta viewed from front. There is an aneurysm below the origin of the renal arteries, ending before the aortic bifurcation. (b) Open abdominal aorta viewed from behind. The aneurysm has been opened revealing a large intraluminal thrombus. Atherosclerotic aneurysms are usually located in the lower part of the abdominal aorta between the renal arteries (above) and the iliac arteries (below). Male, 68 years.
(c,d) Abdominal aortic aneurysm rupturing into the inferior vena cava.
(c) Diagram of the abdominal aorta and the inferior vena cava. The two vessels have joined by a rupture of the aorta into the inferior vena cava. (d) Pulmonary artery containing two crystals of cholesterol, indicating that the pulmonary artery had received contents of the aortic aneurysm.

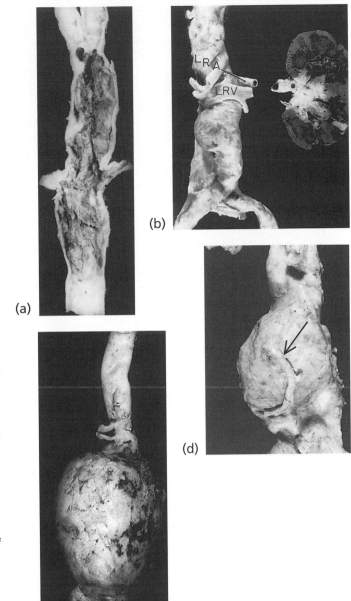

(a)

(b)

(d)

(c)

Figure 177 (a,b) Thrombosis of the abdominal aorta; cases with and without aneurysms of abdominal aorta.
(a) Abdominal aorta without aneurysm formation. There is extensive thrombosis of the aorta both above and below the renal arteries. (b) Abdominal aorta with aneurysm formation and left kidney. The upper level of the aortic aneurysm corresponds to the origin of the left renal artery. The latter is occluded by a thrombus and associated with an infarction of the left kidney. LRV, left renal vein; LRA, left renal artery.
(c,d) Relationship between the origin of the inferior mesenteric artery and the aortic aneurysm.
(c) Large aortic aneurysm viewed from the front. (d) View from the right side. The inferior mesenteric artery is shown arising at the level of the aortic aneurysm (arrow). Male, 52 years.

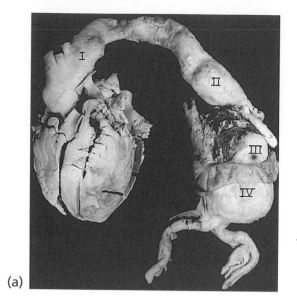

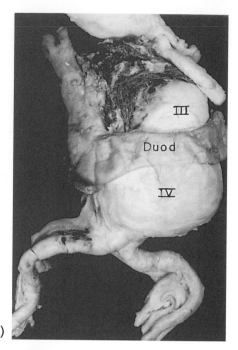

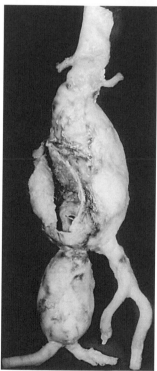

Figure 178 (a,b) Varying location of abdominal aneurysms.
(a) The heart and entire aorta are shown. Four aneurysms (numbered I–IV) are shown. (b) The relationship of the duodenum (Duod) to the classical aneurysm of the abdominal aorta (IV). Erosion of the aneurysm into the duodenum may result in massive GI bleeding.

(c) Variations in abdominal aortic aneurysm.
Atherosclerotic aneurysm of the aorta and right common iliac arteries.

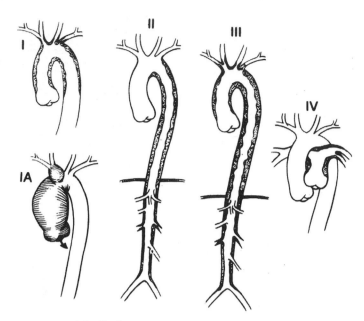

Figure 179 Vasculitis: variation and distribution.
Aortitis types I–III. The bold areas indicate involvement of the vascular wall by chronic inflammation. In type IV there is vasculitis of the pulmonary trunk.
Reprinted with permission from Stehbens and Lie [128].

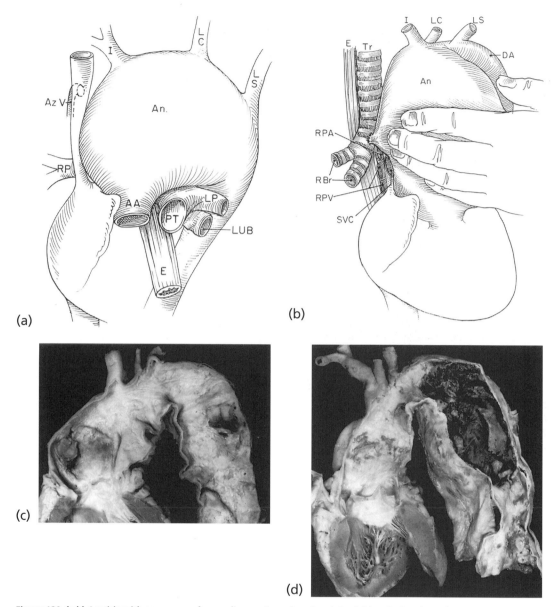

Figure 180 (a,b) Aortitis with aneurysm of ascending aorta and rupture into right mainstem bronchus.
Male, 58 years. Sudden death. (a) View from front. There is a large ascending and aortic arch aneurysm type I (see Figure 179). The arch vessels are unaffected. (b) View from the right side. The aneurysm has eroded into the right mainstem bronchus.
(c,d) Variations of aneurysm of thoracic aorta.
(c) The thoracic aorta as shown is dilated and aneurysmal in the ascending portion and slightly so in the upper descending aorta. Female, 64 years. (d) The descending aorta is aneurysmal. The lumen is filled with clot. Male, 81 years.

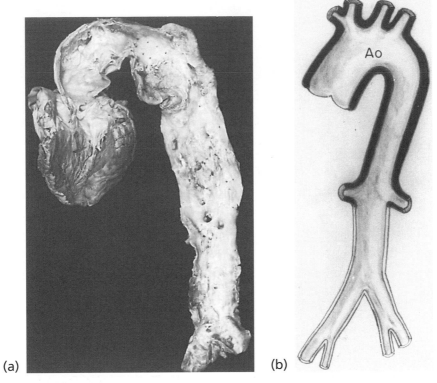

(a)   (b)

Figure 181 Aortitis: "reverse coarctation."
(a) Left ventricle and aorta. There is extensive atherosclerosis causing narrowing of the branches of the aortic arch. Male, 77 years. (b) The aorta showing major thickening of the proximal aorta and proximal branches. Because of branch vessel stenosis the pressure in the lower extremities is higher than that measured in the upper extremities.

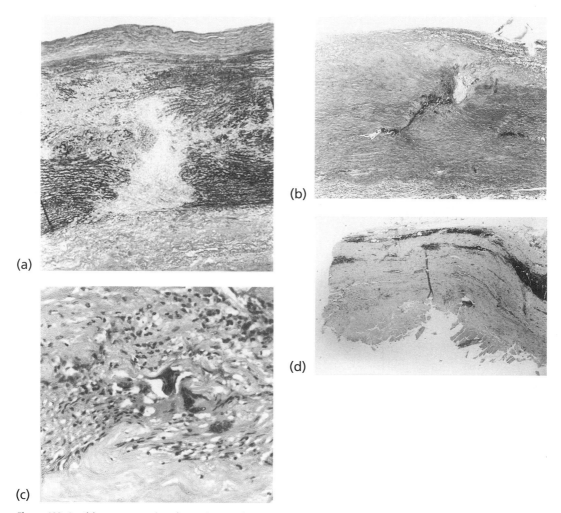

Figure 182 Aortitis: representative photomicrographs.
(a,b) Aorta showing foci of medial interruption. (c) Aortic media with leukocytes and giant cells. (d) Scarring of entire wall of aorta from a prior inflammatory state.

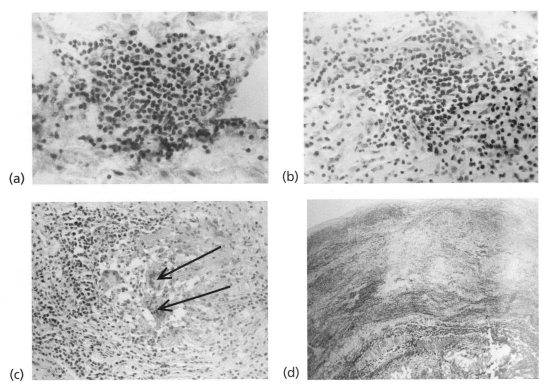

Figure 183 Aortitis: representative photomicrographs.
(a,b) Heavy medial lymphocytic infiltrate. The infiltrate is nonspecific and could represent aortitis from many different causes. (c) Giant cells, (arrows) in addition to leukocytes. (d) Clear zone in the aortic wall suggests cystic medial necrosis.

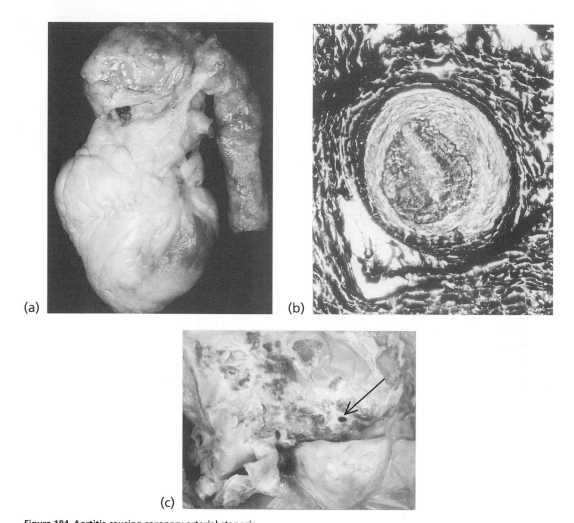

(a)

(b)

(c)

Figure 184 Aortitis causing coronary arterial stenosis.
(a) Heart and thoracic aorta in syphilitic aortitis. There is a large aneurysm of the ascending aorta and aortic arch. (b) A coronary artery with major intimal proliferation in a case of syphilitic aortitis. (c) Opened aortic root. A coronary a ostium (arrow) is narrowed by associated intimal proliferation secondary to chronic inflammation of the aorta.

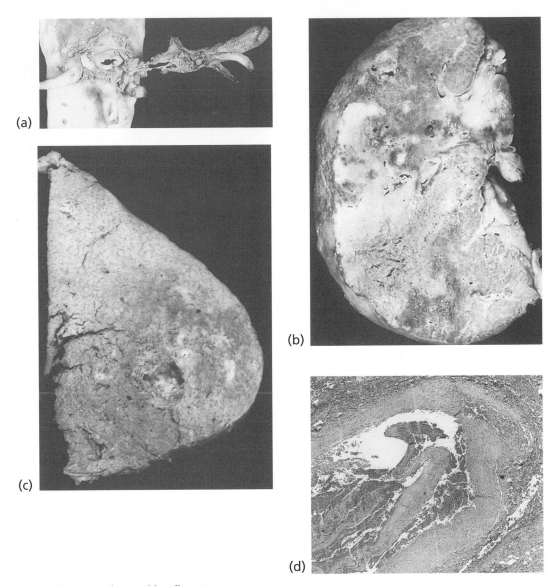

Figure 185 Suppurative arteritis: celiac artery.
Female, 76 years. (a) Celiac artery arising from aorta showing acute inflammation. (b) Splenic infarction. (c) Focal infarction of liver with multiple abscesses. (d) Splenic artery. Acute arteritis with suppurative thrombosis.

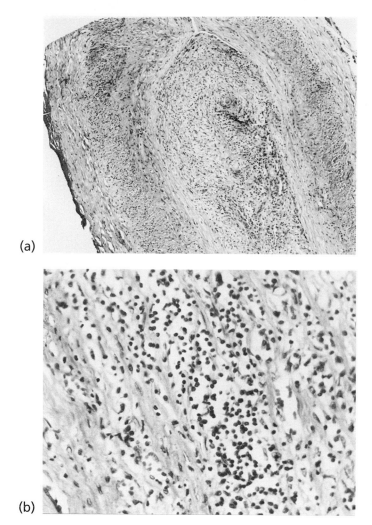

(a)

(b)

Figure 186 Temporal arteritis.
(a) Major intimal leukocytic infiltration in a temporal artery. (b) Temporal arteritis with major granulomatous inflammation of the media.

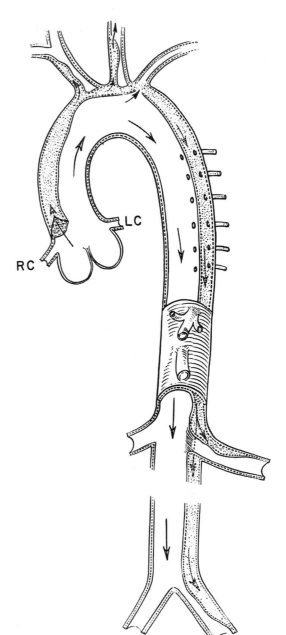

Figure 187 Aortic dissection (dissecting aneurysm of the aorta).
Diagrammatic view of classical aortic dissection involving the full length of the aorta. After a tear of the aortic media (in this instance, the ascending aorta) the path of blood within the wall of the media has the following tendencies: in the ascending aorta, the channel is on the right side; in the aortic arch, the channel is superior; and in the thoracic and abdominal aorta, the channel tends to lie on the left side of the aorta. In this way, the left intercostal arteries are commonly affected, while the right intercostal arteries are usually not disturbed. In the abdominal aorta a false channel tends to lie to the left; this means that the left kidney is more likely than the right to be infarcted. Arteries that arise anteriorly, such as the celiac and mesenteric vessels, tend to be spared from the dissection.

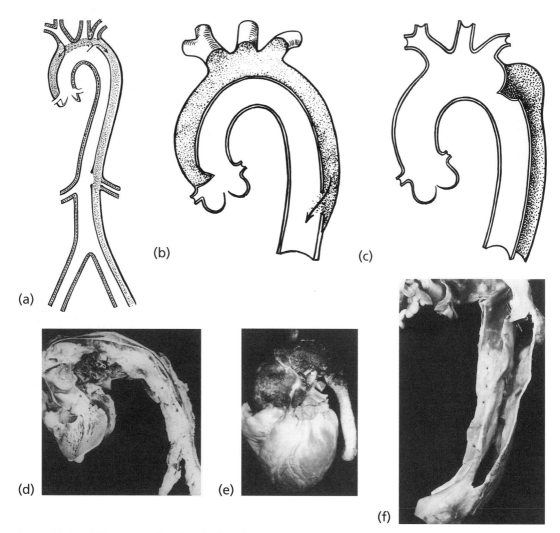

Figure 188 (a,b,c) Three categories of aortic dissection.
(a) Type I involves almost the entire aorta. (b) Type II. The dissection is in the proximal aorta and may or may not involve the branches of the aortic arch. (c) Type III. The dissection begins in the upper descending aorta.
(d) Cases illustrating the three types of aortic dissection.
Type I. (e) Type II. (f) Type III. All three types of aortic dissections may be associated with sudden cardia death.

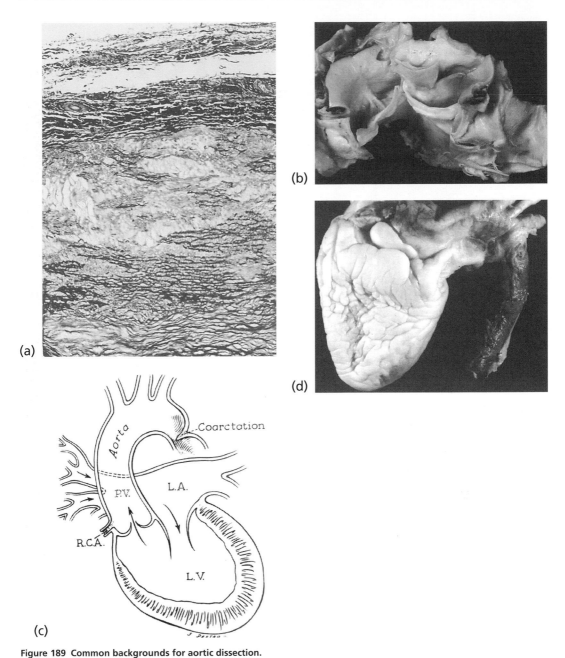

Figure 189 Common backgrounds for aortic dissection.
(a) Photomicrograph of the aorta. There is cystic medial necrosis of aorta with disruption of the elastic fibers in the media. Male, 53 years. (b) Congenital bicuspid aortic valve with the primary tear in the ascending aorta just above the valve. Male, 54 years. (c) Coarctation of aorta. A common precursor to aortic dissection by its association with both hypertension and bicuspid aortic valve. (d) External view of the heart and thoracic aorta. There is a dissection with adventitial hemorrhage present. Chronic systemic hypertension is probably the leading cause of aortic dissection.

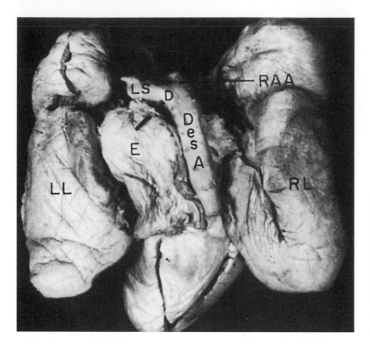

Figure 190 Arterial-esophageal fistula with sudden death.
View of the thoracic organs from behind. There is a right aortic arch (RAA). The black probe shows the path of continuity between the lumens of the descending aorta (Des A) and the esophagus (E). LS, left subclavian; LL, left lung; RL, right lung.
Reprinted with permission from Edwards et al. [131].

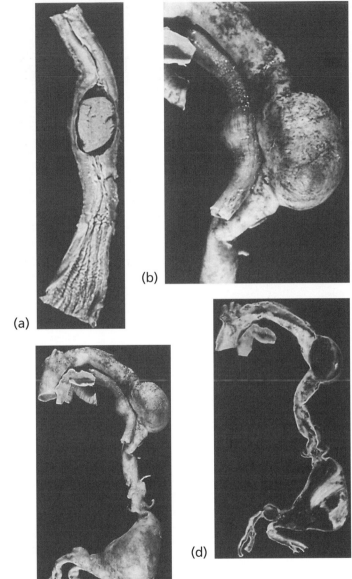

Figure 191 Pulsion diverticulum and aortic aneurysm: potential for aortic-esophageal fistula.
Pulsion diverticulum of esophagus as a precursor to rupture of aorta into esophagus. Female, 88 years.
(a) Opened esophagus with pulsion diverticulum seen in cut section.
(b) Thoracic aorta and attached esophagus showing pulsion diverticulum of esophagus (left) coinciding with position of aortic aneurysm (right). (c) Entire aorta showing pulsion diverticulum of esophagus coinciding with position of thoracic aortic aneurysm. There is also a large abdominal aortic aneurysm.
(d) Interior view of aneurysms. Entire aorta sectioned without the esophagus.

CHAPTER 10

Diseases of the pericardium

The normal pericardium envelops the heart. As in all serous cavities, there is a parietal and a visceral layer. The reflection of these two layers is related to the great vessels. Anteriorly, the reflection is between the aortic valve and the origin of the innominate artery. The reflection on the pulmonary artery is situated near the bifurcation of the arterial structure. The reflections on the superior and inferior vena cava lie near the heart. Pericardial disease may cause symptoms or may be relatively asymptomatic. Various disorders can result in sudden death.

Inflammatory pericardial diseases

There are many causes and types of inflammatory pericardial diseases. Among the types are fibrinous, hemorrhagic, and suppurative. In the abnormal pericardium, healing may be affected by adhesions, chronic effusion, and granulomas. Calcification may impede healing and lead to chronic constrictive pericarditis [132].

In cases with hemorrhagic pericarditis, the etiology may be either fibrinous pericarditis with secondary hemorrhage or hemorrhage as a primary manifestation. Hemorrhage into the pericardium may result from acute myocardial infarction with myocardial rupture, cardiac surgery, aortic dissection with aortic rupture, or accidental injury to the pericardium and great vessels. Saner and associates [133] indicated that pericarditis may be the early manifestation of aortic dissection; this occurs when the primary tear of the aorta lies in the ascending aorta (the intrapericardial segment of the aorta).

Cholesterol pericarditis

Cholesterol pericarditis is a rare disorder of unknown etiology. Stanley and associates [134] report a case of a patient who had recurrent pericardial cholesterol effusions over many years and died with calcific pericarditis 40 years after the onset.

Uremic pericarditis

In patients with end-stage renal disease, pericarditis may be a common manifestation. In some cases, cardiac tamponade may occur. The primary causes of cardiac tamponade in uremic patients, in the order of decreasing frequency, are (1) pericardial effusion usually of the serosanguineous type, (2) massive hemorrhage into the pericardial sac, and (3) collagenization of pericardial exudates by the process of organization. Cardiac tamponade, which may be life threatening, is more common in dialyzed patients than in nondialyzed ones; nevertheless, cardiac tamponade may be observed in nondialyzed patients with end-stage renal disease. Baldwin and Edwards [135] showed that when dialysis is not employed, uremic pericarditis is usually a preterminal event and is characterized by serofibrinous exudation of an amount inadequate to cause cardiac tamponade.

Chronic nonspecific adhesions and effusions of the pericardium

In many instances, the primary cause of chronic pericardial effusions and adhesions is unknown. Categorization of effusions and adhesions is based on the biochemical characteristics of the effusion. The progression from benign effusion to cardiac tamponade depends upon the volume of the effusion, the rate of arrumulation. And the physical characteristics of the pericardiac.

Myocardial abscess leading to diffuse suppurative pericarditis

A myocardial abscess may lead to acute suppurative pericarditis. Infection of an esophageal diverticulum may also lead to suppurative inflammation of the pericardium. Patients who are chronically immunosuppressed may be at increased risk for this rare manifestation of pericardial disease.

Metastatic neoplasms of the pericardium

The pericardium may be a common site for the occurrence of metastatic neoplastic disease. In a review of cases of metastatic neoplasms to the pericardium done by Adenle and Edwards [136], about half of the patients with neoplastic involvement had significant preterminal hemodynamic effects. The most common findings were dyspnea on exertion and coexistent pleural effusions. Thoracic radiographs were not helpful unless there was a large pericardial effusion. The suspicion of metastatic carcinoma to the pericardium depends on elevated venous pressure and enlargement of the pericardiac silhouette. Echocardiography will frequently demonstrate pericardial effusions, sometimes with readily apparent masses on the epicardial surface. While any malignant tumor may metastasize to the pericardium, the most common tumors observed are bronchogenic carcinoma and carcinoma of the breast. Metastatic melanoma has a propensity to involve the pericardium. In general, the metastatic carcinomas to the pericardium form bulky masses. Some exceptions are cases with relatively small amounts of tumor and large volume of effusion. Rarely, the tumors are small.

Chronic constrictive pericarditis

Classically, chronic constrictive pericarditis involves fibrosis and calcification of pericardial tissue. The constriction impairs cardiac filling and reduces cardiac output. As the etiology of constriction has shifted away from infectious causes to other disorders, many cases present now with fibrosis without significant pericardial calcification. Because of the growth of cardiac surgery and the inevitable injury to the pericardium that occurs at the time of operation, many late cases of constriction are now observed in postoperative patients. The physiology of constriction remains the same. The patients have high venous pressure usually with hepatic congestion and ascites. The treatment is surgical, as shown in some of the illustrations. The fragments removed at operation can be overwhelmingly numerous. Sudden death is uncommon in chronic constrictive pericarditis but can occur.

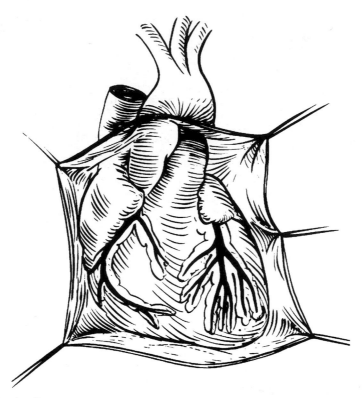

Figure 192 Normal pericardium.
The parietal pericardium has been retracted to show the visceral pericardium and its reflections. Note that the pulmonary trunk and ascending aorta are intrapericardial.

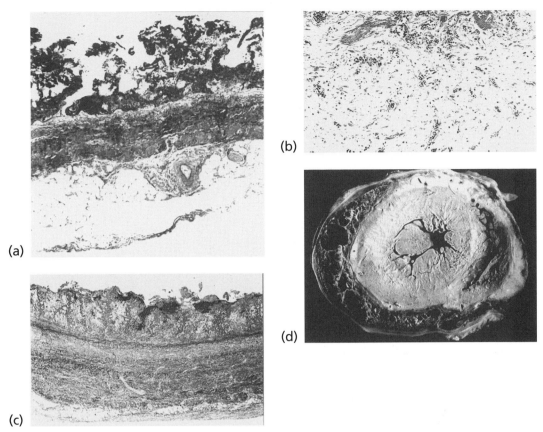

Figure 193 Organization of blood in the pericardium.
(a) Unorganized blood clot on the surface of the visceral pericardium. Female, 58 years. (b) Fibrinous pericarditis undergoing organization. Male, 70 years. (c) Organization of pericardial exudate is yet to be completed. (d) Gross specimen. A thick layer of blood lies between the visceral and parietal pericardium, resulting in cardiac tamponade and sudden death.

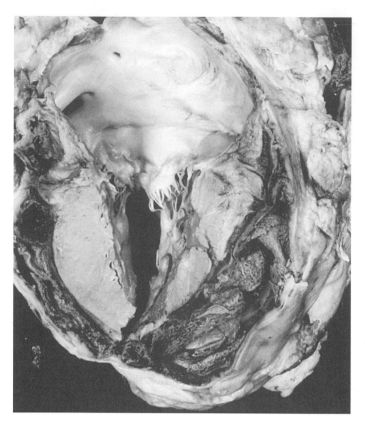

Figure 194 Organization of blood in the pericardium.
Gross specimen of heart and pericardium. Hemopericardium, the result of end-stage uremic pericarditis. There is extensive left ventricular hypertrophy.

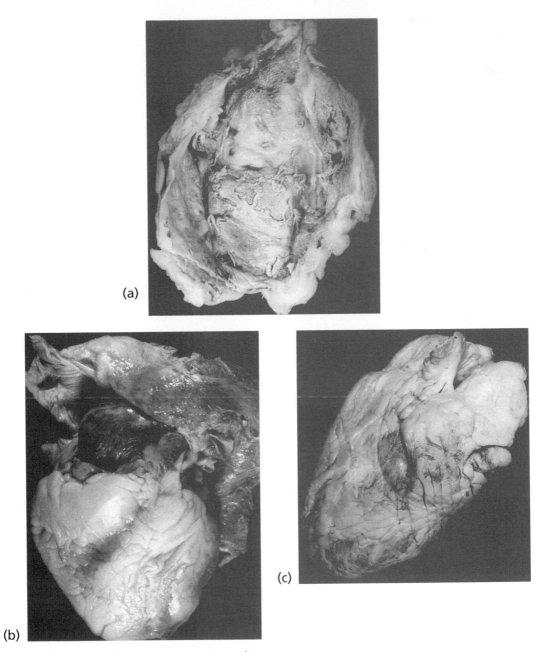

Figure 195 Hemopericardium: spontaneous or traumatic.
(a) Hemopericardium from rupture of ascending aorta in a case of aortic dissection. There may have been leakage into the pericardium before exsanguinating hemorrhage, as the hemorrhage is undergoing organization. Female, 58 years. (b) Rupture of the ascending aorta in case of acute aortic dissection. (c) Right ventricular rupture sustained during an airplane crash. Male, 28 years.

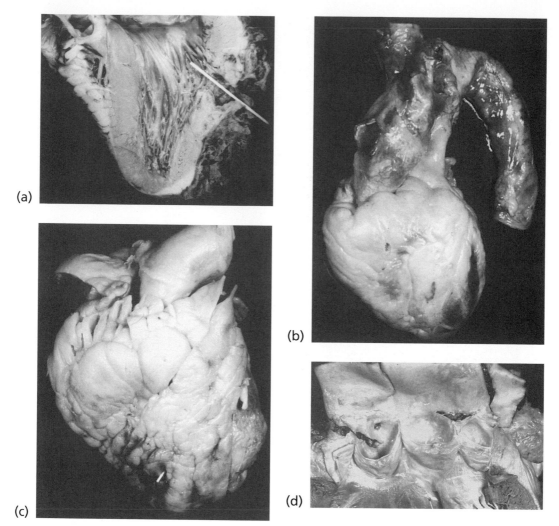

(a)

(b)

(c)

(d)

Figure 196 Hemopericardium with pericardial tamponade and sudden death: spontaneous or traumatic.
(a) Acute myocardial infarction with rupture of left ventricle (probe) and acute cardiac tamponade. Male, 42 years.
(b) Rupture of senile dilatation of the ascending aorta of female, 85 years. (c) Perforation of the right ventricle by cardiac catheter (probe). (d) Two lacerations of the proximal ascending aorta above the aortic valve secondary to recent trauma.

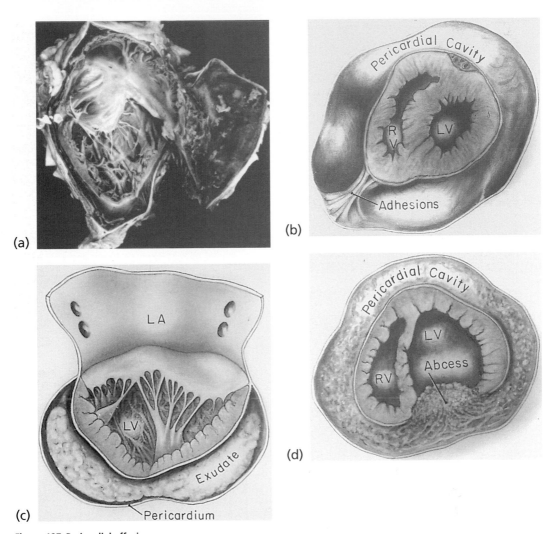

Figure 197 Pericardial effusions.
(a) Gross specimen of the heart and pericardium with the right ventricle open. There is a serous effusion in the pericardium that separates the visceral and parietal layers. (b) Chronic serous effusion with adhesions. (c) Purulent exudate in the pericardium. (d) Heart showing abscess of myocardium with secondary pericardial infection.

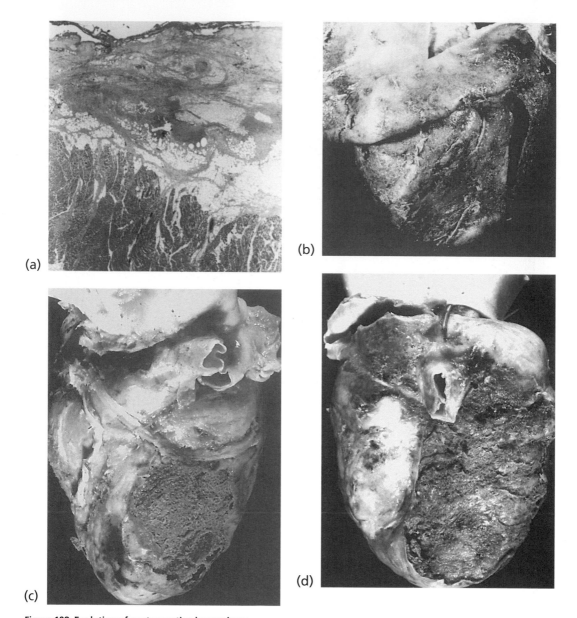

(a)

(b)

(c)

(d)

Figure 198 Evolution of postoperative hemorrhage.
(a) Postoperative hemorrhage can start as fibrinous pericarditis, as seen in this photomicrograph. (b) Postoperative fibrinous pericarditis. Ultimately, the exudate may become hemorrhagic. Male, 70 years. (c,d) Two views showing pericardial hemorrhage starting as fibrinous pericarditis in a patient recovering from recent cardiac surgery. Female, 53 years.

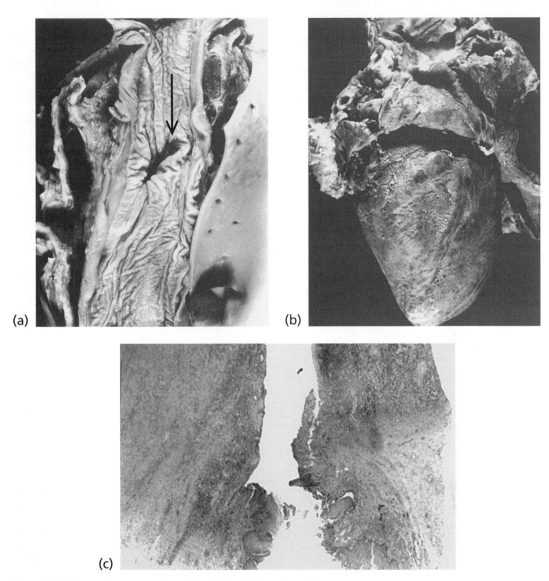

Figure 199 Pericarditis secondary to rupture of diverticulum of esophagus.
Male, 27 years. (a) Interior of esophagus showing proximal opening of esophageal diverticulum (arrow). (b) Surface of visceral pericardium showing acute suppurative pericarditis. (c) Low-power photomicrograph of tract leading from esophagus to pericardium.

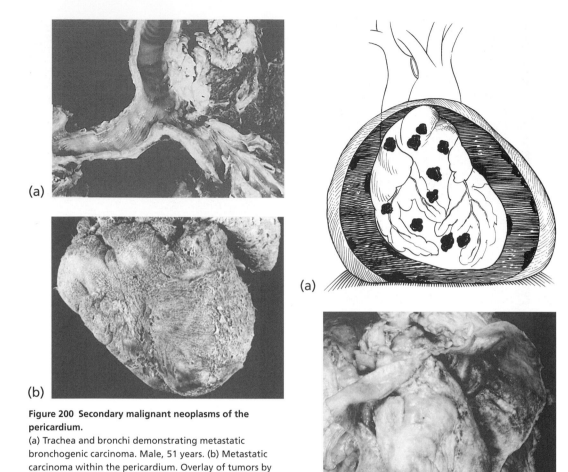

(a)

(b)

(a)

(b)

Figure 200 Secondary malignant neoplasms of the pericardium.
(a) Trachea and bronchi demonstrating metastatic bronchogenic carcinoma. Male, 51 years. (b) Metastatic carcinoma within the pericardium. Overlay of tumors by fibrinous pericarditis is common as a reaction to the pericardial irritation.

Figure 201 Nodular carcinoma with effusion.
(a) Diagrammatic representation of nodules of metastatic carcinoma, shown by black circles, affiliated with massive pericardial effusion. (b) Metastatic bronchogenic carcinoma with localized metastatic nodules. There was a large pericardial effusion separating the visceral and parietal layers of the pericardium. Male, 59 years.

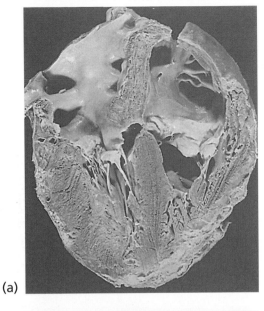

(a)

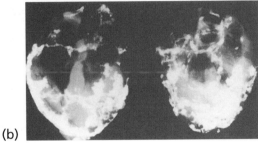

(b)

Figure 202 Classical calcific constrictive pericarditis.
Male, 76 years. (a) Photograph of specimen of heart
showing thickening of pericardium associated with
calcification. (b) Radiograph of specimen of heart shown in
(a) demonstrating distribution of calcification in the
pericardium.
Reprinted with permission from Edwards [109].

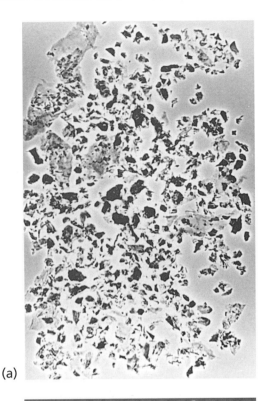

(a)

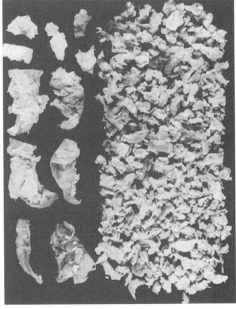

(b)

**Figure 203 Two examples of calcific lesions of pericardium
removed surgically.**
(a,b) The two cases shown are of separate patients with
chronic calcific constrictive pericarditis from which the
lesions were removed surgically. The illustrations portray
the tedious surgery required for removal of such lesions
piece by piece.

CHAPTER 11

Multi-organ system diseases

There are many conditions involving multiple-organ systems that are capable of causing sudden death. In some cases the cardiac system is the site of the primary disorder; in other cases extra cardiac disease presents with secondary cardiac involvement.

Corrected congenital heart disease with sudden death years after operation

The mechanism of sudden death in patients after operation for congenital heart disease varies from case to case and includes late surgical complications, arrhythmias, cardiac failure, progressive pulmonary hypertension, and infectious complications. Some examples are reviewed.

Inadequate myocardial protection at the time of cardiac surgery

The cause of myocardial necrosis varies from lack of oxygen supply due to underlying disease to inadequate myocardial protection during cardiac surgical procedure. Cases have been observed in which the cardioplegia used at the time of cardiac surgery was chemically imbalanced and resulted in major myocardial injury. When this occurs, patients may be unable to be weaned from cardiopulmonary bypass. The gross picture is that of major, dark-red discoloration of the myocardium.

Carcinoid heart disease

The carcinoid tumor has a great tendency to occur either in the bronchus or the ileum. When metastases develop in the liver, fibrotic lesions may occur in the pulmonary valve, the tricuspid valve, and the linings of the right-sided chambers of the heart. Deviation from this pattern is seen rarely but may occur

in individuals with a patent foramen ovale and a right-to-left shunt. In such patients, the carcinoid lesion may also affect the left-sided valves [137]. Similar lesions affecting the right-sided valves may be observed by the administration of the diet drug fenfluramine-phentermine ("fen-phen") [138].

Pritchett and coworkers observed that patients taking pergolide mesylate for Parkinson's disease and restless leg syndrome may also developed the lesions like those seen in carcinoid heart syndrome [139].

Lupus erythematosus

In the autoimmune disease systemic lupus erythematosus, the kidneys may play a major role in lesions recognized by a proliferation of the cells of the renal glomerulus [140]. Associated with renal change are inflammatory lesions of the lung. Valvular involvement is the most common form of heart disease in lupus erythematosus [141]. The classical lesions are the Libman-Sacks vegetations. The mitral valve is most frequently involved with fibrinous vegetations occurring on both the atrial and ventricular surface of the valve. Valvular involvement may lead to severe mitral regurgitation. Mitral stenosis is rare but does occur. The occurrence of coronary atherosclerosis in the absence of other predisposing factors may be seen in patients with lupus erythematosus [142–144]. According to Asanuma et al. [145], the prevalence of coronary artery atherosclerosis is elevated and the age of onset is reduced in patients with lupus erythematosus. Aldoboni et al. [146] reported on a case of lupus erythematosus with primary coronary dissecting aneurysm.

Myocarditis in lupus erythematosus has been reported and considered to be of urgent clinical attention to avoid progression to arrhythmias and conduction disturbances. Dilated cardiomyopathy and heart failure may result [147]. The literature reports the occurrence of congenital complete heart block in children of mothers with lupus erythematosus [49,143].

Lupus erythematosus may be associated with pericarditis and pericardial effusion leading to cardiac tamponade [148] and, rarely, sudden death.

Hypereosinophilic syndrome (Löffler's syndrome)

In the rare condition of hypereosinophilic syndrome, the tricuspid and mitral valves are affected indirectly with the tendency for thrombosis of the endocardium of the right and left ventricles. The "creeping" thrombosis of the ventricular endocardium may eventually entrap the mitral and tricuspid leaflets, binding them to their respective walls of the ventricle [149].

Periarteritis nodosa

Periarteritis nodosa is a systemic necrotizing vasculitis of medium-sized arteries causing ischemia and infarction of affected tissue and organs.

Lesions of the small mesenteric arteries may be associated with segmental infarction of the intestine [150]. The opinion was expressed that these lesions of the small mesenteric arteries are frequently responsible for the majority of cases of so-called nonocclusive infarction of the intestine. Gastrointestinal involvement in periarteritis nodosa is common [151].

There are many cases in which the arterial lesion is restricted to one body system. Periarteritis nodosa may involve the male or female reproductive systems only [152]. Periarteritis nodosa may present with polymyositis [153]. Cutaneous polyarteritis nodosa may be seen as an example of the arterial lesion involving one body system [154]. Subarachnoid hemorrhage is reported from ruptured anterior cerebral arterial aneurysm caused by periarteritis nodosa [155].

Cardiac involvement in patients with primary skeletal myopathies and neuropathies

Various inherited skeletal myopathies and neuropathies can be associated with coexistent cardiomyopathy [156]. Common among these are Becker's muscular dystrophy and Duchenne's muscular dystrophy. Both X-linked disorders affect the dystrophin gene and result in skeletal and cardiac muscle dysfunction. Cardiac fibrosis is common, and conduction in the atrioventricular node is often affected. While Becker's muscular dystrophy tends to have a later age of onset and more mild skeletal symptoms, the cardiac dysfunction is often severe and includes atrial arrhythmias, high-grade heart block and biventricular dilatation with congestive heart failure. The mechanism of death for these affected patients is often either congestive heart failure or an arrhythmia.

Myotonic dystrophy may affect the cardiovascular system, but for most patients the cardiac involvement is mild. In those with cardiac involvement, left ventricular function may be reduced and fibrosis affecting the conduction may be observed.

Friedreich's ataxia is an autosomal recessive neuromuscular disorder that frequently results in cardiac hypertrophy. In about 50% of affected patients the heart resembles that of hypertrophic cardiomyopathy. Sometimes there is extensive intimal coronary artery proliferation without atherosclerosis. Cardiac causes of death are common in these patients.

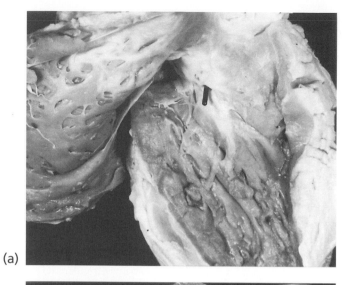

(a)

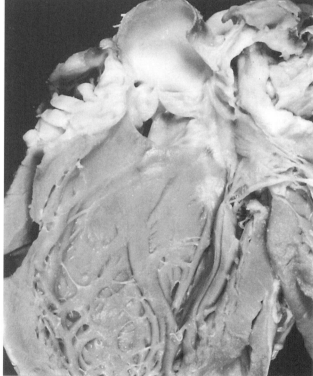

(b)

Figure 204 Operated congenital heart disease with sudden death years after operation.
(a) Partial closure of ventricular septal defect. A small defect remains (probe). Sudden death. (b) View of left ventricle demonstrating a residual ventricular septal defect in the membranous septum. Sudden death. Female, 22 years.

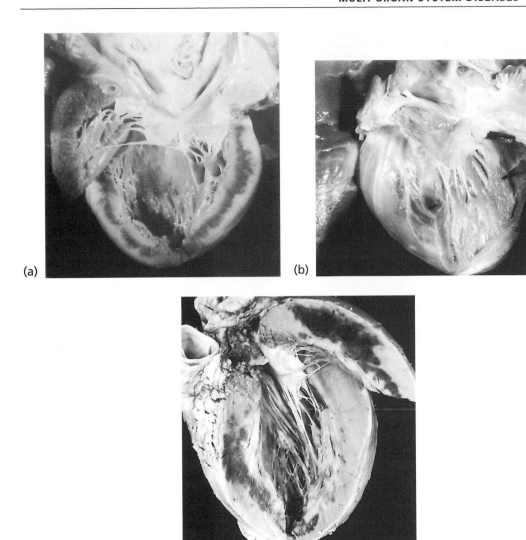

(a)

(b)

(c)

Figure 205 Inadequate intraoperative myocardial protection with myocardial necrosis.
(a,b) Sites of inadequate perfusion shown as dark areas in each ventricle. Male, 8 weeks.
(c) Major discoloration of the myocardium as a result of inadequate myocardial preservation during cardiac operation.
Male, 39 years.

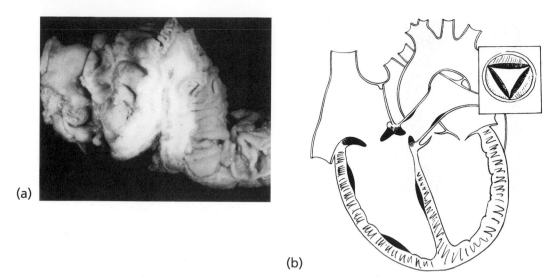

(a)

(b)

Figure 206 Carcinoid heart disease.
(a) Surgically resected ileum with classical carcinoid tumor. (b) Diagrammatic representation of carcinoid heart disease.
The illustration shows pulmonary stenosis with tricuspid valve insufficiency. There is endocardial thickening of the right
ventricle, commonly seen in carcinoid heart disease.
Reprinted with permission from Edwards [109].

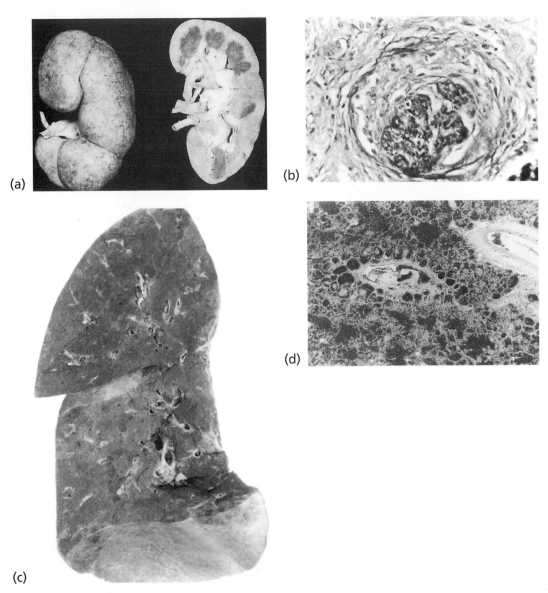

Figure 207 Lupus erythematosus.
(a) Gross specimen of the kidneys demonstrating small cortical hemorrhage. Female, 37 years. (b) A glomerulus showing a proliferation of the capsule. Female, 37 years. (c) Lung showing hemorrhagic discoloration. (d) Photomicrograph of a bronchus showing hemorrhagic foci. Male, 42 years.
Reprinted with permission from Lynch and Edwards [51].

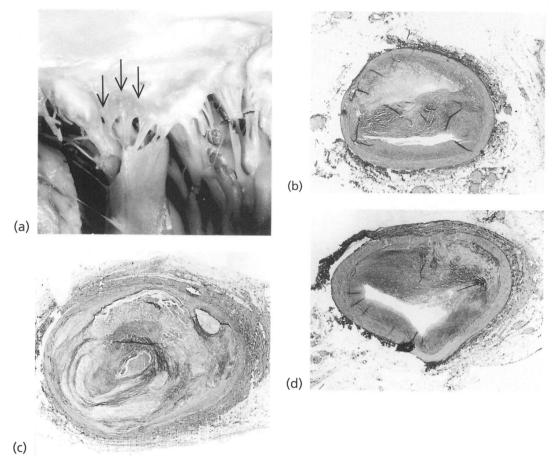

(a)

(b)

(c)

(d)

Figure 208 Coronary atherosclerosis and myocardial infarction associated with systemic lupus erythematosus.
Tsakraklides and associates reported an association between lupus erythematosus and coronary atherosclerosis. Death
was the result of an acute myocardial infarction associated with extensive coronary atherosclerosis in a 29-year-old
woman with systemic lupus erythematosus. None of the recognized underlying causative factors for premature
atherosclerosis were present. (a) Mitral valve. Liebman-Sacks endocarditis. Shallow vegetations characteristic of lupus
erythematosus (arrows). (b) Premature coronary atherosclerosis occurring in a patient with systemic lupus erythematosus.
(c) Coronary atherosclerosis with thrombosis. Patients with systemic lupus erythematosus may exhibit a prothrombotic
tendency. (d) Atherosclerosis of a coronary artery in a patient with lupus.
Reprinted with permission from Tsakraklides et al. [176].

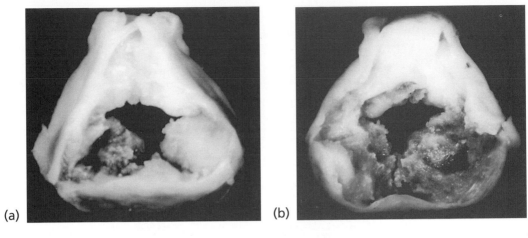

(a)

(b)

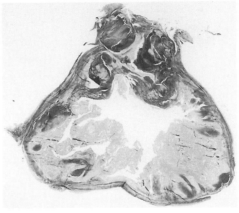

(c)

Figure 209 Aortic valve and lupus erythematosus.
Aortic valve; the cusps are thickened by thrombotic material that encroaches on the lumen. Pritzker and associates reported two cases of aortic stenosis in lupus erythematosus, one in a male and one in a female. The aortic stenosis was caused by fibrocalcific alteration of the aortic valve. (a,b) Surgically excised aortic valves viewed from below. There is fibrocalcific proliferation and ulceration resulting in aortic stenosis. (c) Low-power photomicrograph of the aortic valve showing encroaching of the lumen by fibrocalcific material.
Reprinted with permission from Pritzker et al. [178].

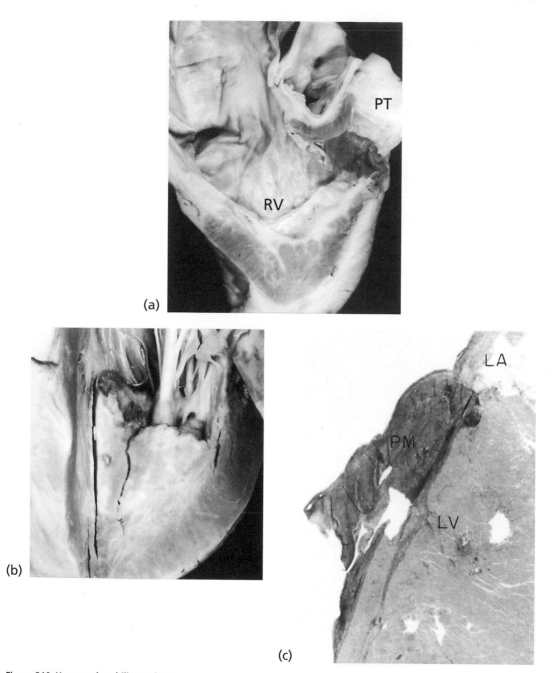

Figure 210 Hypereosinophilic syndrome.
(a) Right side of heart showing endocardial fibrosis and extensive thrombus of the right ventricle (RV), which incorporates the elements of the tricuspid valve. (b) Left side of heart showing mural thrombosis of the left ventricle. The latter encroaches upon the mitral chordae. (c) Photomicrograph of the left ventricle (LV), left atrium (LA) mitral valve area. The posteromedial leaflet of the mitral valve (PM) is incorporated by the reactive tissue, which is characteristic of hypereosinophilic syndrome.
Reprinted with permission from Hall et al. [149].

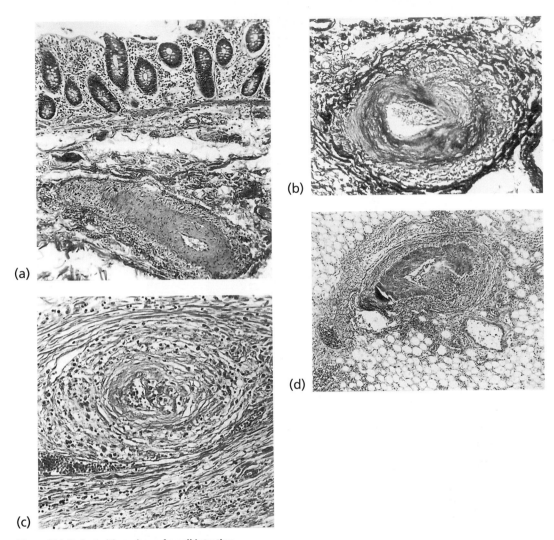

Figure 211 Periarteritis nodosa of small intestine.
Female, 77 years. (a) Small intestine; inflamed artery is present in the serosa. (b) A small artery in the intestine shows the irregularly distributed necrosis. (c) Small artery contains a major inflammatory reaction. (d) A mesenteric artery showing focal necrosis and thrombosis.

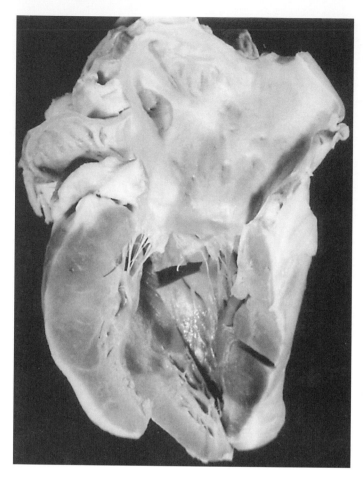

Figure 212 Restrictive cardiomyopathy. Left side of heart showing left ventricular hypertrophy and left atrial dilatation in consistant with Friedreich's ataxia. Male, 15 years.

References

1 Vlodaver Z, Edwards JE. Pathology of coronary atherosclerosis. *Prog Cardiovasc Dis.* 1971;**14**:256.

2 Lecomte D, Fornes P, Nicolas G. Stressful events as a trigger of sudden death: a study of 43 medico-legal autopsy cases. *Forensic Sci Int.* 1996;**79**:1.

3 Prieto A, Eisenberg J, Thakur RK. Nonarrhythmic complications of acute myocardial infarction. *Emerg Med Clin North Am.* 2001;**19**:397.

4 Anderson MW, Christensen NA, Edwards JE. Hemopericardium complicating myocardial infarction in the absence of cardiac rupture. Report of three cases. *Arch Intern Med.* 1952;**90**:634.

5 Van Tassel RA, Edwards JE. Rupture of heart complicating myocardial infarction. Analysis of 40 cases including nine examples of left ventricular false aneurysm. *Chest.* 1972;**61**:104.

6 Edwards BS, Edwards WD, Edwards JE. Ventricular septal rupture complicating acute myocardial infarction: identification of simple and complex types in 53 autopsied hearts. *Am J Cardiol.* 1984;**54**:1201.

7 Vlodaver Z, Edwards JE. Rupture of ventricular septum or papillary muscle complicating myocardial infarction. *Circulation.* 1977;**55**:815.

8 Farmery AD, Chambers PH, Banning AP. Delayed rupture of the mitral valve complicating blunt chest trauma. *Emerg Med J.* 1998;**15**:422.

9 Srichai MB, Casserly IP, Lever HM. Cardiac tamponade masking clinical presentation and hemodynamic effects of papillary muscle rupture after acute myocardial infarction. *J Am Soc Echocardiogr.* 2002;**15**:1000.

10 Bruschi G, Agati S, Iorio F, et al. Papillary muscle rupture and pericardial injuries after blunt chest trauma. *Eur J Cardiothor Surg.* 2001;**20**:200.

11 Simmers TA, Meijburg HW, de la Riviere AB. Traumatic papillary muscle rupture. *Ann Thorac Surg.* 2001;**72**:257.

12 Vlodaver Z, Coe JI, Edwards JE. True and false left ventricular aneurysms. Propensity for the latter to rupture. *Circulation.* 1975;**51**:567.

13 Gobel FL, Visudh-Arom K, Edwards JE. Pseudoaneurysm of the left ventricle leading to recurrent pericardial hemorrhage. *Chest.* 1971;**59**:23.

14 de Boer HD, Elzenga NJ, de Boer WJ, et al. Pseudoaneurysm of the left ventricle after isolated pericarditis and *Staphylococcus aureus* septicemia. *Eur J Cardiothorac Surg.* 1999;**15**:97.

15 Lee PJ, Spencer KT. Pseudoaneurysm of the left ventricular free wall caused by tumor. *J Am Soc Echocardiogr.* 1999;**12**:876.

16 Dubel HP, Rutsch W, Bohm J, et al. Huge false aneurysm of left ventricular posterior wall following resection of an aneurysm of the left ventricular posterior wall. *Catheter Cardiovasc Interv.* 1999;**46**:509.

17 Isner JM, Roberts WC. Right ventricular infarction complicating left ventricular infarction secondary to coronary heart disease. *Am J Cardiol.* 1978;**42**:885.

18 Cohn JN, Guiha NH, Broder MI, et al. Right ventricular infarction – clinical and hemodynamic features. *Am J Cardiol.* 1974;**33**:209.

19 Noren GH, Raghib G, Moller JH, et al. Anomalous origin of the left coronary artery from the pulmonary trunk with special reference to the occurrence of mitral insufficiency. *Circulation.* 1964;**30**:171.

20 Edwards JE, Gladding TC, Weir AB Jr. Congenital communication between the right coronary artery and the right atrium. *J Thor Surg.* 1958;**35**:662.

21 Mahowald JM, Blieden LC, Coe JI, et al. Ectopic origin of a coronary artery from the aorta. Sudden death in 3 of 23 patients. *Chest.* 1986;**89**:668.

22 Steinberger J, Lucas RV Jr, Edwards JE, et al. Causes of sudden unexpected cardiac death in the first two decades of life. *Am J Cardiol.* 1996;**77**:992.

23 Tuna IC, Bessinger FB, Ophoven JP, et al. Acute angular origin of left coronary artery from aorta: an unusual cause of left ventricular failure in infancy. *Pediatr Cardiol.* 1989;**10**:39.

24 Gunning MG, Williams IL, Jewitt DE, et al. Coronary artery perforation during percutaneous intervention: incidence and outcome. *Heart.* 2002;**88**:495.

25 Edwards JE. The coronary vessels in sudden death and in acute myocardial infarction. *Arch Inst Cardiol Mex.* 1980;**50**:383.

26 Ishikawa Y, Sekiguchi K. Akasaka Y, et al. Fibromuscular dysplasia of coronary arteries resulting in myocardial

infarction associated with hypertrophic cardiomyopathy in Noonan's syndrome. *Hum Pathol.* 2003;**34**: 282.

27 Lee AH, Gray PB, Gallagher PJ. Sudden death and regional left ventricular fibrosis with fibromuscular dysplasia of small intramyocardial coronary arteries. *Heart.* 2000;**83**:101.

28 Ropponen KM, Alafuzoff I. A case of sudden death caused by fibromuscular dysplasia. *J Clin Pathol.* 1999;**52**:541.

29 Ogawa T, Nomura A, Komatsu H, et al. Fibromuscular dysplasia involving coronary arteries – a case report. *Angiology.* 1999;**50**:153.

30 Burke AP, Farb A, Tang A, et al. Fibromuscular dysplasia of small coronary arteries and fibrosis in the basilar ventricular septum in mitral valve prolapse. *Am Heart J.* 1997;**134**:282.

31 Imamura M, Yokoyama S, Kikuchi K. Coronary fibromuscular dysplasia presenting as sudden infant death. *Arch Pathol Lab Med.* 1997;**121**:159.

32 Shinohara T, Tanihira Y. A patient with Kawasaki disease showing severe tricuspid regurgitation and left ventricular dysfunction in the acute phase. *Pediatr Cardiol.* 2003;**24**:60.

33 Chesler E, Mitha AS, Edwards JE. Congenital aneurysms adjacent to the anuli of the aortic and/or mitral valves. *Chest.* 1982;**82**:334.

34 Smith TP, Crisera RV, Smisson DC, Edwards JE. Subaortic aneurysm of the left ventricle. *Am J Cardiovasc Pathol.* 1987;**1**:405.

35 Claudon DG, Claudon DB, Edwards JE. Primary dissecting aneurysm of coronary artery. A cause of acute myocardial ischemia. *Circulation.* 1972;**45**:259.

36 Edwards JE. Primary dissection of coronary artery. *Cardiovasc Dis Chest Pain.* 1988;**4**:3.

37 Tveter KJ, Edwards JE. Calcified aortic sinotubular ridge: a source of coronary ostial stenosis or embolism. *J Am Coll Cardiol.* 1988;**12**:1510.

38 Maron BJ, Long L, Moller JH, et al. Cardiomyopathies characterized by evidence of resistance to left ventricular inflow. *Cathet Cardiovasc Diagn.* 1980;**6**:29.

39 Fernando Guadalajara J, Vera-Delgado A, Gaspar-Hernandez J, et al. Echocardiographic aspects of restrictive cardiomyopathy: their relationship with pathophysiology. *Echocardiography.* 1998;**15**:297.

40 Maron BJ, Roberts WC, Edwards JE, et al. Sudden death in patients with hypertrophic cardiomyopathy: characterization of 26 patients without functional limitation. *Am J Cardiol.* 1978;**41**:803.

41 Maron BJ, Edwards JE, Henry WL, et al. Asymmetric septal hypertrophy (ASH) in infancy. *Circulation.* 1974;**50**:809.

42 Lobo FV, Heggtveit HA, Butany J, et al. Right ventricular dysplasia: morphological findings in 13 cases. *Can J Cardiol.* 1992;**8**:261.

43 Bramlet DA, Edwards JE. Congenital aneurysm of left atrial appendage. *Br Heart J.* 1981;**45**:97.

44 Titus JL, Edwards JE. Calcification in myocardial infarcts. *Hum Pathol.* 1989;**20**:721.

45 Raggi P. Coronary-calcium screening to improve risk stratification in primary prevention. *J La State Med Soc.* 2002;**154**:314.

46 Whitehead SJ, Berg CJ, Chang J. Pregnancy-related mortality due to cardiomyopathy: United States, 1991–1997. *Obstet Gynecol.* 2003;**102**:1326.

47 Ibarra-Perez C, Korns ME, Edwards JE. Mesothelioma of the atrioventricular node. *Chest.* 1973;**63**:824.

48 Segal EL, Broadbent JG, Edwards JE. Cardio-aortic fistulas complicating bacterial endocarditis in a case of calcific aortic stenosis. *Proc Staff Meet Mayo Clin.* 1958;**33**: 209.

49 Buyon JP, Friedman DM. Autoantibody-associated congenital heart block: the clinical perspective. *Curr Rheumatol Rep.* 2003;**5**:374.

50 Lynch RP, Edwards JE. Pathologic aspects of systemic hypertension. *Minn Med.* 1964;**47**:24.

51 Lynch RP, Edwards JE. Hypertensive cardiovascular disease: pathological aspects. *Cardiovasc Clin.* 1969;**1**:14.

52 Hanson TP, Edwards BS, Edwards JE. Pathology of surgically excised mitral valves. One hundred consecutive cases. *Arch Pathol Lab Med.* 1985;**109**:823.

53 Edwards WD, Peterson K, Edwards JE. Active valvulitis associated with chronic rheumatic valvular disease and active myocarditis. *Circulation.* 1978;**57**:181.

54 Ben-Shachar G, Vlodaver Z, Joyce LD, et al. Mural thrombosis of the left atrium following replacement of the mitral valve. *J Thor Cardiovasc Surg.* 1981;**82**:595.

55 Edwards JE. Heart failure: the pathologist's view. *Bull Mpls Heart Inst.* 1988;**6**:3.

56 Ozkutlu S, Zyabakan C, Saraclar M. Can subclinical valvitis detected by echocardiography be accepted as evidence of carditis in the diagnosis of acute rheumatic fever? *Cardiol Young.* 2001;**11**:255.

57 Edwards JE. Floppy mitral valve syndrome. *Cardiovasc Clin.* 1987;**18**:249.

58 Perloff JK, Child JS, Edwards JE. New guidelines for the clinical diagnosis of mitral valve prolapse. *Am J Cardiol.* 1986;**57**:1124.

59 Salazar AE, Edwards JE. Friction lesions of ventricular endocardium. Relation to chordae tendineae of mitral valve. *Arch Pathol.* 1970;**90**:364.

60 Chesler E, King RA, Edwards JE. The myxomatous mitral valve and sudden death. *Circulation.* 1983;**67**:632.

61 Edwards JE, Burchell HB. Endocardial and intimal lesions (jet impact) as possible sites or origin of murmurs. *Circulation.* 1958;**18**:946.

62 Osmundson PJ, Callahan JA, Edwards JE. Ruptured mitral chordae tendineae. *Circulation.* 1961;**23**:42.

63 Phillips MR, Daly RC, Schaff HV, et al. Repair of anterior leaflet mitral valve prolapse: chordal replacement versus chordal shortening. *Ann Thorac Surg.* 2000;**69**:25.

64 Arosemena E, Moller JH, Edwards JE. Scarring of the papillary muscles in left ventricular hypertrophy. *Am Heart J.* 1967;**74**:446.

65 Phillips JH, Burgh GE, DePasquale NP. The syndrome of papillary muscle dysfunction. Its clinical recognition. *Ann Intern Med.* 1963;**59**:508.

66 Phillips JH, DePasquale NP, Burch GE. The electrocardiogram in infarction of the anterolateral papillary muscle. *Am Heart J.* 1963;**66**:338.

67 Vlodaver Z, Edwards JE. Mitral insufficiency in subjects 50 years of age or older. *Cardiovasc Clin.* 1973;**5**:149.

68 Davachi F, Moller JH, Edwards JE. Diseases of the mitral valve in infancy. An anatomic analysis of 55 cases. *Circulation.* 1971;**43**:565.

69 Redfield MM, Nicholoson WJ, Edwards WD, et al. Valve disease associated with ergot alkaloid use: echocardiographic and pathologic correlations. *Ann Intern Med.* 1992;**117**:50.

70 Atar S, Jeon DS, Luo H, et al. Mitral annular calcification: a marker of severe coronary artery disease in patients under 65 years old. *Heart.* 2003;**89**:161.

71 Edwards JE. The spectrum and clinical significance of tricuspid regurgitation. *Pract Cardiol.* 1980;**6**:86.

72 Dounis G, Matasakas E, Poularas J, et al. Traumatic tricuspid insufficiency: a case report with a review of the literature. *Eur J Emerg Med.* 2002;**9**:258.

73 Moainie SL, Guy TS, Plappert T, et al. Correction of traumatic tricuspid regurgitation using the double orifice technique. *Ann Thorac Surg.* 2002;**73**:963.

74 RuDusky BM, Cimochowski G. Traumatic tricuspid insufficiency – a case report. *Angiology.* 2002;**53**:229.

75 Messika-Zeitoun D, Thomson H, et al. Medical and surgical outcome of tricuspid regurgitation caused by flail leaflets. *J Thorac Cardiovasc Surg.* 2004;**128**:296.

76 Pereira J, Oliver JM, Mateos M, et al. Tricuspid insufficiency and interatrial septum rupture: a cause of persistent systemic hypoxemia after blunt chest trauma. *J Am Soc Echocardiogr.* 2000;**13**:64.

77 Tanaka S, Kirohashi K, Uenishi T, et al. Surgical repair of a liver injury in a patient: accompanied with tricuspid regurgitation. *Hepatogastroenterology.* 2003;**50**:523.

78 Peterson MD, Roach RM, Edwards JE. Types of aortic stenosis in surgically removed valves. *Arch Pathol Lab Med.* 1985;**109**:829.

79 Edwards JE. The congenital bicuspid aortic valve. *Circulation.* 1961;**23**:485.

80 Castaneda-Zuniga WR, Nath PH, Zollikofer C, et al. Mycotic aneurysm of the aorta. *Cardiovasc Intervent Radiol.* 1980;**3**:144.

81 Feigl D, Feigl A, Edwards JE. Mycotic aneurysms of the aortic root. A pathologic study of 20 cases. *Chest.* 1986;**90**:553.

82 Fukuda T, Hawley RL, Edwards JE. Lesions of conduction tissue complicating aortic valvular replacement. *Chest.* 1976;**69**:605.

83 Wang K, Gobel F, Gleason DF, et al. Complete heart block complicating bacterial endocarditis. *Circulation.* 1972;**46**:939.

84 Edwards JE. Lesions causing or simulating aortic insufficiency. *Cardiovasc Clin.* 1973;**5**:127.

85 Read RC, Thal AP. Surgical experience with symptomatic myxomatous valvular transformation (the floppy valve syndrome). *Surgery.* 1966;**59**:173.

86 Carter JB, Sethi S, Lee GB, Edwards JE. Clinicopathologic correlations. Prolapse of semilunar cusps as causes of aortic insufficiency. *Circulation.* 1971;**43**:922.

87 Carlson RG, Lillehei CW, Edwards JE. Cystic medial necrosis of the ascending aorta in relation to age and hypertension. *Am J Cardiol.* 1970;**25**:411.

88 Simula DV, Edwards WD, Tazelaar HD, et al. Surgical pathology of carcinoid heart disease: a study of 139 valves from 74 patients spanning 20 years. *Mayo Clin Proc.* 2002;**77**:139.

89 Segal EL, Broadbent JC, Edwards JE. Cardioaortic fistulas complicating bacterial endocarditis in a case with calcific aortic stenosis. *Proc Mayo Clin.* 1958;**33**:209.

90 Thell R, Martin FH, Edwards JE. Bacterial endocarditis in subjects 60 years of age and older. *Circulation.* 1975;**51**:174.

91 Becker AE, Becker MJ, Caudon DG, et al. Surface thrombosis and fibrous encapsulation of intravenous pacemaker catheter electrode. *Circulation.* 1972;**46**:409.

92 Cook RJ, Orszulak TA, Nkomo VT, et al. Aspergillus infection of implantable cardioverter-defibrillator. *Mayo Clin Proc.* 2004;**79**:549.

93 Waller BF, Knapp WS, Edwards JE. Marantic valvular vegetations. *Circulation.* 1973;**48**:644.

94 Eliot RS, Kanjuh VI, Edwards JE. Atheromatous embolism. *Circulation.* 1964;**30**:611.

95 Takahashi T, Konta T, Nishida W, et al. Renal cholesterol embolic disease effectively treated with steroid pulse therapy. *Intern Med.* 2003;**42**:1206.

96 Khan AM, Jacobs S. Trash feet after coronary angiography. *Heart.* 2003;**89**:e17.

97 Ghilardi G, Massaro F, Gobatti D, et al. Temporary spinal cord stimulation for peripheral cholesterol embolism. *J Cardiovasc Surg (Torino).* 2002;**43**:255.

98 Ott P, Marcus FI, Sobonya RE, et al. Cardiac sarcoidosis masquerading as right ventricular dysplasia. *Pacing Clin Electrophysiol.* 2003;**26**:1498.

99 Shiraishi J, Tatsumi T, Shimoo K, et al. Cardiac sarcoidosis mimicking right ventricular dysplasia. *Circ J.* 2003;**67**:169.

100 Kato Y, Morimoto S, Uemura A, et al. Efficacy of corticosteroids in sarcoidosis presenting with atrioventricular block. *Sarcoidosis Vasc Diffuse Lung Dis.* 2003;**20**:133.

101 Kasai H, Suzuki J, Imamura H, et al. A case of cardiac sarcoidosis with advanced atrioventricular block. Failure of endomyocardial biopsy diagnosis and success in detecting. *Heart Vessels.* 2003;**18**:50.

102 Duke C, Rosenthal E. Sudden death caused by cardiac sarcoidosis in childhood. *J Cardiovasc Electrophysiol.* 2002;**13**:939.

103 Okura Y, Dec GW, Hare JM, et al. A clinical and histopathologic comparison of cardiac sarcoidosis and idiopathic giant cell myocarditis. *J Am Coll Cardiol.* 2003;**41**:322.

104 Josselson AJ, Pruitt RD, Edwards JE. Amyloid localized to the heart. Analysis of twenty-nine cases. *Arch Pathol.* 1952;**54**:359.

105 Yomtovian RA, Walley VM, Bollinger RD, et al. Isolated valvular amyloid. *Am J Cardiovasc Pathol.* 1989;**2**:365.

106 Pruitt RD, Daugherty GW, Edwards JE. Congestive heart failure induced by primary systemic amyloidosis: a diagnostic problem. *Circulation.* 1953;**8**:769.

107 Ocel JJ, Edwards WD, Tazelaar HD, et al. Heart and liver disease in 32 patients undergoing biopsy of both organs with implications for heart or liver transplantation. *Mayo Clin Proc.* 2004;**79**:492.

108 Ruttenberg HD, Steidl RM, Carey LS, et al. Glycogen-storage disease of the heart. Hemodynamic and angiocardiographic features in 2 cases. *Am Heart J.* 1964;**67**:469.

109 Edwards JE. Effects of malignant noncardiac tumors upon the cardiovascular system. *Cardiovasc Clin.* 1972;**4**:281.

110 Murphy WR, Carter JB, Lucas RV, et al. Recurrent myxosarcoma of left atrium. *Chest.* 1975;**67**:733.

111 Ibarra-Perez C, Korns ME, Edwards JE. Mesothelioma of the atrioventricular node. *Chest.* 1973;**63**:824.

112 Shrivastava S, Jacks JJ, White RS, et al. Diffuse rhabdomyomatosis of the heart. *Arch Pathol Lab Med.* 1977;**101**:78.

113 Edwards EA, Edwards JE. The effect of thrombophlebitis on the venous valve. *Surg Gynecol Obstet.* 1937;**65**:310.

114 Wellons E, Rosenthal D, Schoborg T, et al. Renal cell carcinoma invading the inferior vena cava: use of a "temporary" vena cava filter to prevent tumor emboli during nephrectomy. *Urology.* 2004;**63**:380.

115 Adams HP Jr. Patent foramen ovale: paradoxical embolism and paradoxical data. *Mayo Clin Proc.* 2004;**79**:15.

116 Horton SC, Bunch TJ. Patent foramen ovale and stroke. *Mayo Clin Proc.* 2004;**79**:79.

117 Menzel T, Kramm T, Wagner S, et al. Improvement of tricuspid regurgitation after pulmonary thromboendarterectomy. *Ann Thorac Surg.* 2002;**73**:756.

118 Sapala JA, Wood MH, Schuhknecht MP, et al. Fatal pulmonary embolism after bariatric operations for morbid obesity: a 24-year retrospective analysis. *Obes Surg.* 2003;**13**:819.

119 Pitto RP, Hamer, H, Fabiani R, et al. Prophylaxis against fat and bone-marrow embolism during total hip arthroplasty reduces the incidence of postoperative deep-vein thrombosis: a controlled, randomized clinical trial. *J Bone Joint Surg Am.* 2002;**84-A**:39.

120 Edwards WD, Edwards JE. Clinical primary pulmonary hypertension: three pathologic types. *Circulation.* 1977;**56**:884.

121 Anderson JL, Durnin RE, Ledbetter MK, et al. Pulmonary veno-occlusive disease. *Am Heart J.* 1979;**97**:233.

122 Edwards BS, Weir EK, Edwards WD, et al. Coexistent pulmonary and portal hypertension: morphologic and clinical features. *J Am Coll Cardiol.* 1987;**10**:1233.

123 Butto F, Lucas RV Jr, Edwards JE. Pulmonary arterial aneurysm. A pathologic study of five cases. *Chest.* 1987;**91**:237.

124 Lowery RC Jr., Ergin MA, Galla J, et al. Successful treatment of multiple simultaneous great vessel disruptions. *Ann Thorac Surg.* 1986;**41**:672.

125 Fernandez Guerrero ML, Aguado JM, Arribas A, et al. The spectrum of cardiovascular infections due to Salmonella enterica: a review of clinical features and factors determining outcome. *Medicine.* 2004;**83**:123.

126 Sanchez-Recalde A, Mate I, Merino JL, et al. Aspergillus aortitis after cardiac surgery. *J Am Coll Cardiol.* 2003;**41**:152.

127 Choi JB, Yang HW, Oh SK, et al. Rupture of ascending aorta secondary to tuberculous aortitis. *Ann Thorac Surg.* 2003;**75**:1965.

128 Stehbens WE, Lie JT, eds. *Vascular Pathology.* London: Chapman and Hall; 1995:623–653.

129 Younge BR, Cook BE Jr, Bartley GB, et al. Initiation of glucocorticoid therapy: before or after temporal artery biopsy? *Mayo Clin Proc.* 2004;**79**:483.

130 Edwards WD, Leaf DS, Edwards JE. Dissecting aortic aneurysm associated with congenital bicuspid aortic valve. *Circulation.* 1978;**57**:1022.

131 Edwards BS, Edwards WD, Connolly DC, et al. Arterial-esophageal fistulae developing in patients with anomalies of the aortic arch system. *Chest.* 1984;**86**:732.

132 Ford EJ, Bear PA, Adams RW. Cholesterol pericarditis causing cardiac tamponade. *Am Heart J.* 1991;**122**:877.

133 Saner HE, Gobel FL, Nicoloff DM, et al. Aortic dissection presenting as pericarditis. *Chest.* 1987;**91**:71.

134 Stanley RJ, Subramanian R, Lie JT. Cholesterol pericarditis terminating as constrictive calcific pericarditis.

Follow-up study of patient with 40 year history of disease. *Am J Cardiol.* 1980;**46**:511.

135 Baldwin JJ, Edwards JE. Uremic pericarditis as a cause of cardiac tamponade. *Circulation.* 1976;**53**:896.

136 Adenle AD, Edwards JE. Clinical and pathologic features of metastatic neoplasms of the pericardium. *Chest.* 1982;**81**:166.

137 Simula DV, Edwards WD, Tazelaar H, et al. Surgical pathology of carcinoid heart disease: a study of 139 valves from 75 patients spanning 20 years. *Mayo Clin Proc.* 2002;**77**:139.

138 Connolly HM, Crary JL, McGoon MD, et al. Valvular heart disease associated with fenfluramine-phentermine. *N Eng J Med.* 1997;**337**:581.

139 Pritchett AM, Morrison JF, Edwards WD, et al. Valvular heart disease in patients taking pergolide. *Mayo Clin Proc.* 2002;**77**:1280.

140 Proven A, Bartlett RP, Moder KG, et al. Clinical importance of positive test results for lupus anticoagulant and anticardiolipin antibodies. *Mayo Clin Proc.* 2004;**79**:467.

141 Fluture A, Chaudhari S, Frishman WH. Valvular heart disease and systemic lupus erythematosus: therapeutic implications. *Heart Dis.* 2003;**5**:349.

142 Bruce IN, Urowitz MB, Gladman DD, et al. Risk factors for coronary heart disease in women with systemic lupus erythematosus: the Toronto Risk Factor Study. *Arthritis Rheum.* 2003;**48**:3159.

143 Bruce IN, Gladman DD, Ibanez D, et al. Single photon emission computed tomography dual isotope myocardial perfusion imaging in women with systemic lupus erythematosus. II. Predictive factors for perfusion abnormalities. *J Rheumatol.* 2003;**30**:288.

144 Park CW, Shin YS, Kim SM, et al. Papillary muscle rupture complicating inferior myocardial infarction in a young woman with systemic lupus erythematosus and antiphospholipid syndrome. *Nephrol Dial Transplant.* 1998;**13**:3202.

145 Asanuma Y, Oeser A, Shintani AK, et al. Premature coronary-artery atherosclerosis in systemic lupus erythematosus. *N Engl J Med.* 2003;**349**:2407.

146 Aldoboni AH, Hamza EA, Majdi K, et al. Spontaneous dissection of coronary artery treated by primary stenting as the first presentation of systemic lupus erythematosus. *J Invasive Cardiol.* 2002;**14**:694.

147 Wijetunga M, Rockson S. Myocarditis in systemic lupus erythematosus. *Am J Med.* 2002;**113**:419.

148 Cauduro SA, Moder KG, Tsang TS, et al. Clinical and echocardiographic characteristics of hemodynamically significant pericardial effusions in patients with systemic lupus erythematosus. *Am J Cardiol.* 2003;**92**:1370.

149 Hall SW Jr, Theologides A, From AH, et al. Hypereosinophilic syndrome with biventricular involvement. *Circulation.* 1977;**55**:217.

150 Arosemena E, Edwards JE. Lesions of the small mesenteric arteries underlying intestinal infarction. *Geriatrics.* 1967;**22**:122.

151 Levine SM, Hellmann DB, Stone JH. Gastrointestinal involvement in polyarteritis nodosa (1986–2000): presentation and outcomes in 24 patients. *Am J Med.* 2002;**112**:386.

152 Fraenkel-Rubin M, Ergas D, Sthoeger ZM. Limited polyarteritis nodosa of the male and female reproductive systems: diagnostic and therapeutic approach. *Ann Rheum Dis.* 2002;**61**:362.

153 Plumley SG, Rubio R, Alasfar S, et al. Polyarteritis nodosa presenting as polymyositis. *Semin Arthritis Rheum.* 2002;**31**:377.

154 Bauza A, Espana A, Idoate M. Cutaneous polyarteritis nodosa. *Br J Dermatol.* 2002;**146**:694.

155 Takahashi JC, Sakai N, Iihara K, et al. Subarachnoid hemorrhage from a ruptured anterior cerebral artery aneurysm caused by polyarteritis nodosa. Case report. *J Neurosurg.* 2002;**96**:132.

156 Worton, R. Muscular dystrophies: diseases of the dystrophin-glycoprotein complex. *Science.* 1995;**270**:755.

157 Kalke B, Edwards JE. Localized aneurysms of the coronary arteries. *Angiology.* 1968;**19**:460.

158 Gobel FL, Visudh-Arom K, Edwards JE. Pseudoaneurysm of the left ventricle leading to recurrent pericardial hemorrhage. *Chest.* 1971;**59**:23.

159 Joassin A, Edwards JE. Late causes of death after mitral valve replacement. *J Thorac Cardiovasc Surg.* 1973;**65**:255.

160 Gomes AS, Nath PH, Singh A, et al. Accessory flaplike tissue causing ventricular outflow obstruction. *J Thorac Cardiovasc Surg.* 1980;**80**:211.

161 Edwards JE, Burchell HB. Pathologic anatomy of mitral insufficiency. *Mayo Clin Proc.* 1958;**33**:497.

162 Edwards JE. Varieties of valvular heart disease, part I: mitral valvular disease. *Pract Cardiol.* 1982;**8**:111.

163 Edwards JE. Mitral insufficiency resulting from "overshooting" of leaflets. *Circulation.* 1971;**43**:606.

164 Pocock WA, Bosman CK, Chesler E, et al. Sudden death in primary mitral valve prolapse. *Am Heart J.* 1984;**107**:378.

165 Lee KS, Johnson T, Karnegis IN, et al. Acute myocardial infarction with long-term survival following papillary muscular rupture. *Am Heart J.* 1970;**79**:258.

166 Levy MJ, Siegal DL, Wang Y, et al. Rupture of aortic valve secondary to aneurysm of ascending aorta. *Circulation.* 1963;**27**:422.

167 Dry TJ, Edwards JE, Vigran IM, et al. Mycotic aneurysm of the posterior tibial artery complicating subacute bacterial endocarditis. Antemortem diagnosis confirmed by instrumental means. *Proc Mayo Clin.* 1947;**22**:105.

168 Edwards JE. Clinicopathologic correlations. Mitral insufficiency secondary to aortic valvular bacterial endocarditis. *Circulation*. 1972;**46**:623.

169 Becker AE, Becker MJ, Martin FH, et al. Clinicopathologic correlations. Bland thrombosis and infection in relation to intracardiac catheter. *Circulation*. 1972;**46**:200.

170 Waller BF, Knapp WS, Edwards JE. Marantic valvular vegetations. *Circulation*. 1973;**48**:644.

171 Layman TE, Lyne BW, Edwards JE. Systemic amyloidosis with cardiac involvement suggesting coronary arterial disease. *Geriatrics*. 1968;**23**:103.

172 Tiffany FB, Woodburn RL, Edwards JE. Diabetes-nephrosis syndrome and cardiac complication. *Minn Med*. 1963;**46**:1141.

173 Carter JB, Cramer R Jr, Edwards JE. Mitral and tricuspid lesions associated with polypoid atrial tumors, including myxoma. *Am J Cardiol*. 1974;**33**:914.

174 Edwards JE. Bacterial endocarditis and prosthetic valves. *Circulation*. 1973;**47**:3.

175 Edwards WD, Edwards JE. Clinical primary pulmonary hypertension: three pathologic types. *Circulation*. 1977;**56**:884.

176 Tsakraklides VG, Blieden LC, Edwards JE. Coronary atherosclerosis and myocardial infarction associated with systemic lupus erythematosus. *Am Heart J*. 1974;**87**:637.

177 Edwards JE. *An Atlas of Acquired Diseases of the Heart and Great Vessels*. Philadelphia, Pa: WB Saunders; 1961.

178 Pritzker MR, Ernst JD, Caudill C, et al. Acquired aortic stenosis in systemic lupus erythematosus. *Ann Int Med*. 1980;**93**:434.

Index